AGAINST THE TIDE

DEDICATION

To my patients –
they taught me all I know

Against the Tide

Back pain treatment – the breakthrough

An Autobiography

Robin McKenzie
with Ron Bybee

Dunmore Publishing

Published in 2009 by
Dunmore Publishing Ltd
P.O. Box 25080
Wellington
books@dunmore.co.nz
www.dunmore.co.nz

National Library of New Zealand Cataloguing-in-Publication Data
McKenzie, Robin, 1931-
Against the tide : back pain treatment, the breakthrough : an autobiography / Robin McKenzie with Ron Bybee.
ISBN 978-0-958269-26-1
1. McKenzie, Robin, 1931-. 2. Physical therapists—New
New Zealand—Biography. 3. Backache—Physical therapy.
I. Bybee, Ron. II. Title.
615.82092—dc 22

Distributed by
Spinal Publications Ltd
P.O. Box 2026
Raumati Beach 5255
Phone 04 299 7020
Fax 04 299 7010
www.spinalpublications.co.nz

Set in Warnock 11.5/15.5
Designed by Matthew Bartlett

CONTENTS

Commitment

Until one is committed,
there is hesitancy, the chance to draw back,
always ineffectiveness concerning
all acts of initiative and creation

There is one elementary truth
the ignorance of which kills countless ideas
and splendid plans:
that the moment one definitely commits oneself,
then providence moves too.

All sorts of things occur to help one
that would never otherwise have occurred.
A whole stream of events issues
from the decision, raising in one's favour
all manner of unforeseen incidents, which no man
could have dreamed would have come his way.

Whatever you can do or dream you can, begin it.
Boldness has genius, power and magic in it.
Begin it now.

GOETHE

FOREWORD

I am very pleased to offer a foreword for Robin McKenzie's autobiography. It is impossible to overestimate his impact on the non-operative care of the human spine and extremities. This is the compelling story of a man who, by astute observation over many years, developed a previously undefined concept of care and promoted it into medical and physiotherapy circles with extraordinary determination.

Back pain is the most common musculoskeletal ailment; it has no barriers of sex, race, age or geography. Yet, the treatments offered by the "experts" currently include perhaps 20 concepts. Why has the McKenzie method of care survived and grown?

By shrewd observations over 25 years in his physiotherapy practice in New Zealand, McKenzie recognized that particular repeated movements played a remarkable role in being able to change the location of pain. From the medical standpoint this is an absolutely unknown concept, even today. All that is considered necessary is to assess the range of motion of the joint. And then there was the concept of "centralization" of pain. Having the patient repeat particular movements revealed that this process could shift the location of pain from the leg or arm to the low back or neck. McKenzie was the first to understand and develop this process.

In the 1960s, increasingly confident of his ideas and the benefits for patients, McKenzie needed the support and affirmation of colleagues and other medical professionals. He looked outward to the world. He persuaded his wife that they should re-mortgage their home to provide the funds to travel to Europe. Unhappily, his visits to the international back experts left him with enormous doubts and a dilemma. Had he really made one of the most significant discoveries as to the cause and treatment of spine pain, or were his observations just a fluke? Why had clinicians worldwide not drawn the same conclusions, and why had the best of them failed to see what had become so clear to him. The experts had offered him little chance to explain and no support for his ideas. Was it worth sailing against such a strong wind?

There would not have been a book to write if Robin McKenzie had not persevered, as he did – against enormous scepticism and often considerable resistance. Perhaps working in the tiny South Pacific nation of New Zealand, where there were really few powerful forces which could deter him, had actually advantaged him. There he had worked as an independent therapist/businessman. As long as patients derived treatment benefits, more would come. That certainly happened. There were many other modes of care available, such as chiropractic, osteopathy and the usual physical therapy, all of which had advocates and varying degrees of success. And he was working in a field where even success was hard to define. Was success a 24–48-hour fix, or was it – as he came to ardently believe – a process of engagement with the patient that heals and prevents recurrences and thus decreases the incidence of the ubiquitous spinal pain? Still today much that goes under the heading of Physical Therapy has little benefit for patients. Short-term control of pain will not change structure. Ultimately only the active participation of the patient in some sort of progressive exercise programme that is based on rational principles can be justifiably claimed as therapeutic.

My first meeting with McKenzie was by no means planned. He had firmed up his concept and knew it was reliable. He also recognized the need to test its legitimacy outside New Zealand. Serendipitously, one of the physiotherapists working at the spine rehabilitation programme I was directing at Rancho Los Amigos, Los Angeles had heard about this foreign maverick who was treating spine problems differently. At that time most of the experts believed spinal extension (arching backward) was not a beneficial manoeuvre and that abdominal strengthening was the most appropriate treatment programme for acute and chronic back pain. There was no scientific support for this, but a clinician consensus. This visiting physiotherapist from New Zealand was now promoting the rejected possibility of arching backward – and claimed he was achieving significant success. It was suggested we invite McKenzie to evaluate our patients, many of whom were not improving through our chronic programme. McKenzie came. He was initially discouraged by the numbers of patients who had multiple surgeries to the low back and who were still suffering pain and he found many of these patients now impossible to help. Surgical intervention for back pain was less common in New Zealand and his treatment regimen had largely been developed for those who had suffered considerably without successful intervention and who were looking at surgery as a last option. His treatment was generally highly successful and he was soon able to demonstrate in the US that for some of these surgical patients, and many others who had chronic pain but had not had surgery, he could greatly reduce or eliminate their pain.

Encouraged by these patients, by some clinicians, and with my support as well, he proceeded to run educational programmes in the United States. The success of his concepts became more and more apparent to those therapists and physicians willing to step away from familiar yet unproved modes to look at the reality of successful patient recovery.

Robin McKenzie's story is an heroic journey over a professional and personal lifetime. It is important because not only does it identify a testable concept of care, but it draws attention to the many and diverse barriers in modern medicine to effective non-operative musculoskeletal care. When nearly all the "smart people" either ignore you or actively resist a demonstrable assessment and treatment, how do you cope and go forward? There is a lesson here for us all. Careful observation is a worthy basis for the building of new concepts, and rejection does not mean you are wrong. Every scientific breakthrough, from Einstein to Semmelweiss, had early detractors and often only gained acceptance and credibility over time and with determined advocacy.

Although my own meeting with Robin was an unguarded moment many years ago, it resulted in my education in an alternative concept. Today, however, I remain astonished at the continuing determined rejection of this by the experts in this particular area of medicine. The barriers McKenzie has faced in promoting what is a simple and effective treatment option are irrational and extraordinary. The future is bright, however. Scientific support is gathering momentum and there is growing pressure for revision of standards and recommendations for musculoskeletal disorders.

This is a very good story and it engages the reader emotionally in its many moments of suspense, disappointment, humor and triumph. At the end, however, the reader is left puzzling over why the journey that has resulted in relief and cure for so many has been so difficult, yet marveling at the intrepid character of the man who has traveled that hard road.

Vert Mooney
Clinical Professor Orthopaedics Surgery, University of California, San Diego.
Medical Director, Spine and Therapy Centre, San Diego, Ca.
April 2009

NOTE FROM THE CO-AUTHOR

A wise man will make more opportunities than he finds.
SIR FRANCIS BACON

My initial encounter with Robin McKenzie was merely a result of being in the right place at the right time. During the period 1978–80 I was enrolled in an advanced Master's program in the Physical Therapy Department of the University of Southern California. I had been practising for more than ten years at that point and felt that I was a good, orthopedically oriented, physical therapist, having taken coursework that included the teachings of the gurus of the day: Cyriax, Maitland, Kaltenborn, Mennell, Paris, Mulligan, Rocobado, and Grimsby. I believed I was successful with my patients and I was not searching for new approaches to spine problems.

My graduate program at USC was in two parts. There was a year of didactic class work followed by an optional year of specialization in clinical skills. I had chosen the musculoskeletal disorders track. I am not sure that anyone had preceded me in that choice so I was told to organize my own course of specialization using the many resources in the Southern California area.

One of the resources I found was a great therapist named Barbara Stone. She was involved as an officer with an orthopedic special interest group from the greater Los Angeles area. I attended interesting meetings of that group and spent time studying in her clinic. During that time she told me of this physiotherapist from New Zealand who was advocating that we should extend (bend backward) some lumbar spine pain patients. This was a very strange notion to me as I was immersed, along with the majority of my colleagues, in the theories of Dr Paul Williams who advised that all patients with low back pain should be flexed (bent forward). Williams' Flexion Exercises were commonly applied in the clinics of North America. It was, in fact, so common that one of my assistants would frequently say that we had x number of patients referred for 'Willy's Benders' for the week.

Barbara reported that Robin McKenzie was returning to America soon and suggested that I listen to what he had to say. A course was organized by Alice McCleary in San Diego and I was able to register for half tuition on account of my student status. Barbara also arranged for me subsequently to sit in on an 'advanced' McKenzie course in Los Angeles which was attended by practitioners who had been exposed to the McKenzie approach the year earlier.

In San Diego some 30–40 of us were shoe-horned into a small classroom for four days in one of the local medical centres. There was no course outline or manual to assist us in our note taking and there were very few slides to illustrate the lecture portions of the course. We all wrote as rapidly as we could as McKenzie talked to us about his methods of examining and treating patients with low back pain. It was difficult to write down all of the main points discussed as things progressed rapidly. The material was a bit confusing as it was so different and contrary to what we had previously been told by Williams and Dr Rene Cailliet. It seemed that all of the clinics in America had a series of books by Cailliet on the reference shelf. Both doctors recommended flexion (forward bending) for the patients and strongly advised against any exercise or positioning in an extension (backward) direction.

All I was now hearing was so heretical in the light of my previous education that it was hard to accept. Had I received only the description of McKenzie's methods I would likely have dismissed him as another entertaining nutcase looking to separate me from my money and with nothing of worth to teach. However, he treated patients in front of us that were brought to him cold. He knew nothing about them. He would examine them and treat them, with the majority of them improving significantly during that initial visit. McKenzie then had them return over the next days to follow up with them and many were symptom free before the course was completed. One patient was particularly impressive. He was wheeled in on a gurney directly from the Emergency Room. He could not stand because of the intensity of the pain in his back and leg. Within 20 minutes he was up, walking, and smiling as he left. I was intrigued, though still skeptical. This was the most unusual continuing education course I had ever attended, and the success with the patients convinced me that there was truth to be discovered in Robin McKenzie's ideas.

I went home to ponder on what I had seen and heard. When back in the clinic I tried to apply the principles that had been outlined. It was difficult with just my notes to guide me. Some of the patients responded quickly and well, just as they had for McKenzie. Others did not seem to respond at all, and yet others complained of increased pain. For those it seemed easier to fall back on the methods we had used before, and in a busy clinic that was easy to do. But I continued to be fascinated by the rapidity with which some patients improved and by others who experienced complete abolition of symptoms within a few visits. I was further convinced that there was something of great value to be learned.

I continued to search for McKenzie courses and attended them when I could. Each time I listened to him I learned more, and with each patient he demonstrated additional principles of examination and treatment. Initially the format was the same, but with time there were more slides, a course outline and there were always different patients.

I continued in this way for some time. Success with my patients was improving though not universal. I felt at that time that some were 'McKenzie' patients and some were not. (I am saddened that some practitioners are still stuck in that dilemma.) After a time, I was not really satisfied with that position and decided that I must put the method to a definitive trial. I determined that I would apply the method to all of my spine patients and that I would apply the approach as purely as I knew how. There would be no more slipping into whatever was quick and convenient at the moment, I would stick to the principles that McKenzie taught. At that point, we had *Treat Your Own Back* and *The Lumbar Spine: Mechanical Diagnosis and Therapy* as guides, as well as increasingly more complete course manuals and visual aids.

When I began applying the teachings purely, my success with my patients improved incredibly. I kicked myself for not having done it sooner. I had become a disciple.

It was not always easy. At that time I was a therapist in the US military. I was moved frequently and would then have to convince another set of physicians and colleagues that what I was doing was good for the patients and they should let me proceed with what I had to offer. The government was not lenient about what could be included in a patient's chart. In the early days I was not allowed to place a McKenzie assessment form in the chart. Finally, in frustration, I had the forms printed on sticky-backed paper that I could glue to the proper government form. Once it was stuck there, it was impossible to remove and, most importantly, the appropriate government number was visible in the corner. Another issue was that we were required to provide care to all those eligible without cost to them. I knew of the value of the lumbar and cervical rolls and the *Treat Your Own Back* and *Treat Your Own Neck* books so I had to convince the medical supply people wherever I went that it was worth adding these to the tight budget so they could be distributed to the appropriate patients without charge.

As the variety of courses grew I attended them all and, when possible, several times. Spine patients became my primary interest because I knew that we had something to offer them that would result in rapid improvement for the majority of them.

When news of the developing Diploma course in Mechanical Diagnosis and Therapy (MDT) reached me, I knew that I wanted to go to New Zealand to receive advanced training. Dana Greene and I were privileged to be first to be formally trained in that residency course. Upon returning from New Zealand I began the process of training to become faculty for the McKenzie Institute, a position I continue to hold. I actively taught courses for the Institute for ten years and now continue to teach McKenzie principles to my entry-level physical therapy students in the university setting.

Learning and applying the principles of MDT from Robin McKenzie has changed my professional and personal life for the better. Now, 30 years after my introduction to the method, I continue to be amazed by the effectiveness of the application of the method to patients. I feel lucky to have been in Southern California when McKenzie finally had the opportunities to begin to teach the world about the development of his serendipitous discovery years earlier when a patient placed himself in an odd extended position. I am thankful to have had a small part in taking the message to the world.

As I have considered Robin McKenzie's professional life and the insight he has given the world into the complex problems of spinal pain I have been astounded by the story related in this book. One has to think that many of us in today's litigious world of healthcare upon finding a patient in the extremely unorthodox position of spinal extension would have immediately taken him out of the 'dangerous' position, returned him to conventional care, and thanked our lucky stars that he had not been damaged and was not considering a law suit. Treatment consisting of exercise in the opposite direction was the wisdom of the day, especially in North America, and Dr Paul Williams preached strongly against any sort of extension exercise or position. But McKenzie, rather than being relieved that he had ducked a bullet, followed up on the unexpected and positive outcome and after many years of study and experimentation presented us with a method of conservative spinal care which is unique and extremely effective. He has endured years of derision and abuse from professional groups but persisted in his quest to expand his own understanding of the mechanics of the human body. His theories were so advanced that it has taken years for the research community to catch up to his thinking. A vast body of scientific studies now support his concepts. (See Donelson's *Rapidly Reversible Low Back Pain* for a thorough discussion of the literature.)

History is packed with examples of accidental and sagacious discoveries while in pursuit of something else: Christopher Colombus' discovery of America, Alexander Fleming's discovery of penicillin, and Alfred Bernard Nobel's discovery of dynamite are just a few examples. Robin McKenzie's discovery of the relevance of Mr Smith's position to his initial improvement and then recovery was another of these. But what made the difference – and always makes the difference – was this man's desire to understand what he had seen and his recognition of its worth. He had the tenacity to face difficulties throughout the world as he tried to share what he believed was valuable. And it has turned out to be something very good for the entire world.

Robin McKenzie's story needs to be known by a larger part of the world. He has spent his entire professional life trying to improve his and our understanding and treatment of patients suffering from pain and dysfunction related to mechanical problems. The road has not been easy. It has cost him a great deal of personal time and money to get people to listen and to consider his message. He mortgaged his home and left his young family to travel the developed world to seek understanding and share his findings. Publishing his ideas required him to form his own publishing company when others would not help to disseminate his materials. He is the author of six books, has been published in the *New Zealand Medical Journal* and contributed to many texts on spine problems. He has not sought to enrich himself through his discoveries; monies earned have gone back into the McKenzie Institute, which is a charitable trust, and have been used to fund research and education.

As McKenzie's methods have become better known, some have taken note. In 1982 he was made an Honorary Life Member of the American Physical Therapy Association. In 1983 he was elected to membership in the Society for the Study of the Lumbar Spine. In 1984 he became a founding Fellow of the American Back Society and in 1985 he was awarded an Honorary Fellowship of the New Zealand Society of Physiotherapists. In 1987 he was made an Honorary Life Member of the New Zealand Manipulative Therapists Association and in 1990 an Honorary Fellow of the Chartered Society of Physiotherapists in the United Kingdom.

In 2004 the results of a survey of therapists who were members of the Orthopedic Section of the American Physical Therapy

Association were published in the United States. The therapists were asked to identify which physicians or physical therapists of all time they believed had made the biggest impact on their thinking or performance in orthopedic physical therapy. Robin McKenzie was voted as having had the greatest influence of all.

The honors which have pleased him the most came from the Queen. In 1990 he was named: Invested Officer of the Most Excellent Order of the British Empire (OBE). In 2000 he became an Invested Companion New Zealand Order of Merit (CNZM). Robin McKenzie is an extraordinary man who has given much to the world and asked nothing in return except that we are honest and forthright with our words and our patients. It has been a privilege and honor to have played a part in telling his amazing story.

Ron Bybee
DPT, OCS, Dip MDT.
USA

CHAPTER 1

THE EARLY YEARS

In 1930 in the small country town of Masterton (pop. 5,000), New Zealand, Lilian Anderson, a hairdresser, and Robert McKenzie, a lawyer, began a romantic relationship. Apparently not wanting to become a family, but wanting to legitimize the birth of an expected child, the couple – my parents – agreed to marry but to separate immediately after my birth. I was born on 20 April 1931 in Auckland and named Robin Anthony McKenzie. Lilian had gone to Auckland for the birth to avoid the gossip that would abound in the small town.

My mother was a relatively successful women's hairdresser and was determined to run her own life and provide for me. While we did not have a refrigerator or a car, I remember always feeling cared for and safe. If my mother experienced any discrimination due to her chosen independence and solo-parent status in an era when such a choice would not have been readily accepted, I was unaware of it. I did, though, gradually become aware as I grew up that my mother went to considerable lengths to prevent my father contacting or having any relationship with me. She frequently reminded me what a bad person he was and that I should avoid him.

In time I learned that when my mother met my father he was a widower with a 15-year-old daughter, Josephine. He was a respected lawyer attached to the Maori Land Court, which had been established to deal with the settlement of Maori land claims in the 1930s. My father paid my mother a monthly sum to assist in my support, but there was little contact between us, even though for several years I would watch him walking past our front gate every morning on his way to the office. I recall only four or five meetings with him during my childhood, the first being when I was about 10. Now this seems unjust and I have deeply regretted the lack of contact all through my adult life. I came to know later that Mum had kept me away from the entire McKenzie family, many of whom lived in the town and district.

My father's grandfather, Alexander, and his wife, Mary Gollan McKenzie, had emigrated from Scotland to Melbourne in 1852. The family was undoubtedly one of the many victims of the Highland Clearances in Scotland in the first half of that century. Things did not work out well in Australia and in 1854 they sailed to New Zealand on the vessel *Flash,* landing on Petone foreshore in Wellington Harbour.

Upon their arrival in New Zealand the McKenzie family was given a land grant of 41 acres near Masterton in the southern part of the North Island. Four of the five children born to Alexander and Mary, including my grandfather, Roderick McKenzie, grew up and remained in this region. Robert, my father, one of the youngest of 13 children, was born in 1888 in Fernridge, five miles west of Masterton, to Roderick and Elizabeth Harvey McKenzie. Many of his family were involved in farming, but Robert became a lawyer.

Much later I sought more detail about my Scottish heritage and became very proud of it. I remembered seeing my father wearing the highland dress – to me he looked splendid in his kilt, especially when he played the pipes. I wish I had been able to learn more from him about Scotland, as he had been to visit his ancestral origins on several occasions. I eventually found the opportunity to acknowledge my origins by including the McKenzie family crest in the logo of the McKenzie Institute International.

At six weeks of age I was diagnosed with pyloric stenosis, a congenital condition which prevented food from passing from the stomach into the intestine, and in 1931 I was apparently only the second infant in New Zealand to have surgery for this condition. Without the operation I would have died, and I understood from my mother that at the time my recovery was considered quite miraculous. Follow-up surgeries at 15 and 35 years of age to release adhesions from the original surgical procedure were a small price to pay for my good fortune.

This early threat to my life was probably the reason that my mother considered me a bit fragile. I was always conscious of her conviction that I might not cope with anything too physically or intellectually demanding and at one point she encouraged me to take up her own profession – ladies hairdressing. Despite this suggestion, she was concerned about my education and wanted more for me. She was never satisfied with the curricula offered and I was moved from school to school. I actually attended six different primary schools, one of which was a boarding school, Scots College, located in Wellington – four hours away by train. Aged only six, I was so homesick that I was allowed to return to Masterton after only a short stay.

I have many memories of my childhood and youth – some doubtless of formative value and others of the adventures that rural New Zealand, with its relatively safe and certainly beautiful environment, offered its young.

Early in my life I had an experience with the police that helped confirm to me that the world was just and the authorities looked out for those with good intentions. I was about six years old, walking home from school, and a very large boy, one Dib McLachlan, stole two pennies from me. Arriving home, and with my mother at work at the salon, I climbed on a stool to reach the phone and dialed the number of the local policeman to report this serious crime. Later that afternoon Dib came around to return the stolen coins and to apologize to me. This boy would get into much more serious trouble with the local policeman, but he never bothered me again and my faith in the goodness of the system was, for the moment at least, unassailable.

My mother was a very active socialist who belonged to the Labour Party and the Society for Closer Relations with the Soviet Union. She was one of six children from a family of dedicated socialists. They had emigrated to New Zealand from England in 1908 and almost immediately the whole family became active in politics. She would host evenings with like-minded socialists and communists in our house. This was in the years leading up to the Second World War – I would have been about seven or eight. By these activities she acquired something of a reputation in the rather conservative area where we lived.

I remember the announcement of war. I was staying with my mother's sister, Aunt Margaret Thorn, in Thames, further north in the country, when a BBC radio broadcast by Neville Chamberlain, Prime Minister of Great Britain, announced the outbreak of World War II. All the adults were very upset by the news but I, not understanding the gravity of the situation, was most interested in the newsreel at the local "pictures" on Saturday afternoons, which showed the German invasion and the bombing of Holland and Poland. My uncle, Jim Thorn, a Member of Parliament in the first Labour Government, was called to Wellington for urgent consultation. I knew this meant he was a very important person, something I had not previously realized.

But for a young country lad, the war brought excitement – I had little understanding of the tragedy it represented for so many who were caught up in its realities. Many of the families in Masterton and our district were most painfully affected by the war. Their sons, eager for adventure, went willingly off to serve – in the Middle East against the Germans, and later against the Japanese in the Pacific. Many did not return. One family in the town, the Bunnys, lost twin boys in North Africa within two weeks. They were family friends and my mother was very upset.

A number of my relatives were active in the Home Guard, with spotting duties at Castlepoint on the east coast of the North Island where they were charged with watching for the approaching invasion by the Japanese. Fortunately that never eventuated, thanks largely to the presence of the US Marines in the South Pacific.

During the war years a different kind of shattering event occurred in the town, leaving an indelible memory for those who experienced it. In June 1942, when I was 11, the town was rocked by an earthquake which all but destroyed the main shopping avenue. The street became impassable as buildings on both sides collapsed into the roadway. The first quake occurred at 7.50 in the evening, marked for me by a large bowl of fruit falling from a shelf onto my bed. Many people were inside one of the three local movie theatres expecting the films to start. With the first quake, some left. The second, more powerful quake occurred about 10.50 – just after the theatres had closed. This tremor caused the collapse of the roof of one of the buildings. Had it occurred half an hour earlier there would have been many fatalities, but luckily only a few people in the town suffered minor injuries.

There was a very well-provisioned United States Marine camp near town. Could we have been luckier! With my friends I watched enthralled as huge trucks, earth-moving equipment, and all the Marines came into the town as in an invasion. The Marines responded so quickly to the earthquake that in just two days the road had been cleared, the debris removed, and all manner of assistance had been set up for those in need of help with damaged houses and buildings. Their heavy equipment was not a common sight in New Zealand and bulldozers were almost unknown. The Americans worked this machinery almost continuously until the demolition and clean-up was complete. They did a wonderful job, which the town never forgot; the Americans were held in enormously high regard anyway because they had come to New Zealand's aid when it looked as though the Japanese were planning to invade.

We kids frequently hung around the Marines' camp, situated on a small aerodrome at the south end of town. It took us only 15 minutes racing on our bikes to get from home to the camp. The guards at the entrance turned a blind eye to our unauthorized entry and after a few weeks we knew many of these big, friendly men by their unusual names. They chewed gum constantly and gave us packs of it and lots of other great stuff. We wondered why they were so keen to know if we had older sisters.

While there was gasoline rationing during those years, it of course did not affect a family without a car, and although there was also rationing of some foods, particularly meat and butter, the black market seemed to provide whatever people felt that they really needed over and above the rationed amounts. Alcohol was severely limited, but my mother told me that my father still managed to drink a bottle of whiskey every day! I don't know how she knew this with such certainty.

I sometimes wondered if I was a bit of a bother to my mother as I was growing up. Perhaps I limited some of her political and personal activities. In 1945, with the war finally over, and ever looking for a better school for me and perhaps for more personal freedom, Mum enrolled me for my secondary education at Wairarapa College – as a boarder. With the school being just over our back fence I could not understand why I had to be a boarder. I was 14 and perhaps a little rebellious, but as I jumped the fence to home almost every day it was not really like a boarding school at all.

I remember some of the teachers at the college, several of whom were former soldiers who had just returned from the war. I came to understand how very lucky we were to have had those teachers. They had travelled to the other side of the world, fought bloody battles, taken very hard knocks, and lost many good friends. While as children we could never have understood what they had experienced, their stories inspired us and we remembered them and grew through them.

My years at Wairarapa College were for the most part very enjoyable. I had many good friends and I directed much energy to sports. I think now that academically I may have been rather lazy and unfocused. Students were placed in detention or even physically punished if they did not complete their homework assignments and I was frequently in difficulty with my teachers for these reasons. I became very familiar with the pattern on the carpet in the headmaster's office, receiving 'six of the best' where it hurt most fairly regularly.

I was pretty passionate about sport during those years, especially field hockey, which I played for the college Senior Eleven. Another sport, rather outside the school curriculum and certainly outside school hours, was rabbit hunting. An élite squad of us loved it – rabbits were so plentiful in the area around the town and flourished on the river flats. I saved all my pocket money to buy the .22 calibre cartridges for our frequent hunting adventures. We would ride our bikes five or six miles out of town and would bag 40 or 50 rabbits on a Saturday afternoon. We'd often gut the rabbits, hang their entrails in the river close by and wait to shoot the eels that would gather. This was teenage-boy heaven. The ritual included the lighting of a large fire on an island in the middle of the river and sharing the items we each brought to cook for the traditional feast. We would fry bacon and eggs in a pan and throw large potatoes into the fire until they looked like charcoal. We ravenously ate everything – cinders, charcoal and all. On one occasion the fire spread in the wind and caught the scrub on the riverbed. What a wonderful sight it was, the flames roaring up in the air and the smoke going for miles. We were exhilarated by it all, but by hometime began to feel very nervous about the reaction we might receive once back. As it turned out, no one seemed to have noticed, but we avoided repeating the performance.

In those days students needed to attain passing grades on the five major subjects to be eligible to enter university. When it came time for exams my hitherto lack of interest in the academic side of school life resulted in my failing three of the five required subjects. Fortunately the Assistant Principal, Mr Stuart Mills, believed that I had more potential than I had demonstrated. He devoted many hours to tutoring me in the failed subjects. My self-selected mentor was really quite extraordinary. He would take me aside and assure me I could do well. I started to believe him and to my surprise, and I imagine Mr Mills' delight, I then passed all of the certificate subjects the next time around and was accredited for university entrance.

Life was to change now – I had my ticket to the adult world and a future. I had enjoyed a carefree and in many ways charmed childhood and youth with special friends – Peter Lawson, Rex Nichols, David Esau, Randall Thompson, Roger Tristram, John Tristram, Don Shaw,

Brian Shaw, Tony Levien and David Palmer – and I had experienced the kindness and generosity of many adults over those years.

My mother, who never remarried, remained a dedicated socialist – that is until she inherited a considerable sum of money. Earlier, she had responded to a request to go to a local retirement home to provide hairdressing services to the residents. There she became acquainted with Mrs Gillies, a resident, and they became friends. Later, when the home experienced financial difficulties and was forced to close, and Mrs Gillies had no living family and nowhere to live, Mum invited her to come to live in our home. She lived with us for a couple of years and continued living with Mum for several more years after I left home. During that time Mum acquired the previously unaffordable car and refrigerator, and with Mrs Gillies' passing, inherited her estate consisting of £20,000 in cash and a farm. Mum sold the farm in 1956 for more than £100,000, about three years after Mrs Gillies' death. Her lifestyle then improved immeasurably, and during my student years in Dunedin the occasional £30 or £40 came my way – considerably, if temporarily, improving a struggling student's financial wellbeing. Unfortunately Mum's windfall did not last; over time she lost a large proportion of her fortune at the off-course betting shop. Betting on the horses had become something of an obsession with her.

CHAPTER 2

CHOOSING A CAREER

When it came time to consider what to do next, I found my persistent inattention at high school had narrowed my choices. I talked to the vocational guidance officer and thought I might like to study medicine, but quickly learned that my grades would not qualify me for medical school. Well, I had no intention of following my mother's earlier suggestion of a career as a ladies' hairdresser; my new-found pride in my success in the school exams was energizing and I was now determined to go to university.

A friend of my mother, a Miss Olive Sutherland, who was also Head of the English Department at Wairarapa College, suggested I consider physiotherapy. She had heard that it was a new and interesting university degree course. I knew nothing at all about it – it was a new word to my ears – but Miss Sutherland contacted a soldier, Ian Taylor, who had recently returned from overseas duty in the Army and was under the rehabilitation support scheme. He had decided to become a physiotherapist, and his enthusiasm fired me up. Mum clearly had doubts about my going off to university, but her sense of obligation for her friend's efforts on my behalf meant plans were laid.

At the end of the war the Medical School at Otago University in Dunedin was held in high regard. In 1946, with the backing of that school, the university had converted the old Otago Hospital's School of Massage into a School of Physiotherapy. New rehabilitation techniques were being developed throughout the world, prompted by the urgent need to assist and hasten recovery for wounded veterans. The university recognized the need and established the new school to offer professional training in physiotherapy.

It was to this school that I sought entry. Despite my application being late, I was invited to an interview in Wellington with Miss Joan McGrath, the secretary of the Physiotherapy Board. All prospective students of physiotherapy had to undergo an interview with Miss McGrath. She was probably in her mid-fifties, with graying hair – a formidable lady both in bulk and intellect. When she asked me why I wanted to go into physiotherapy I replied that I did not have the marks for Medical School but still wanted to help people with injuries. I hoped this altruism would help me get selected. As my application had been lodged late, it was in fact considered only after another student dropped out, so I was enormously relieved when I was accepted and told I would begin at Otago University in late February 1950.

The people of Dunedin were very proud of their university, which at that time included the only Medical School in the country. The university encouraged commitment to study but also allowed students to broaden their horizons – to find themselves – before going out into the world. I began to feel very excited about the life ahead.

I was far too late to apply for accommodation in a hall of residence, so my mother contacted a Mrs Davidson who lived in Roslyn, a suburb near the university. She agreed to take me as a lodger for six months in place of another student who declined her offer at the last minute. After a couple of weeks there I understood why the vacancy had arisen. Although very kind, Mrs Davidson was a fussy and meticulous housekeeper. I had started to smoke a pipe and she objected strongly to my lighting up inside the house. She was also a teetotaller and wanted everyone else to be so as well. Life was clearly going to be impossible.

By great luck I found another physio student, Hugh Bramwell, seeking somewhere to live. We found a one-room flat in a large old mansion on the hills above the university and with my new-found freedom and a new-found friend, I was set to go. With so much time and so many options in front of me, the idea of serious work seemed of secondary importance. But Hugh had gone through secondary school with flying colors, gaining honours in most of the subjects he took and was of a more responsible and serious disposition. I found his commitment most disconcerting, to say the least. As soon as we arrived home from class, Hugh would go to his desk and review the day's work, whereas I went with Craig Cameron, another physio student, to the Bowling Green Hotel for a few glasses of gin and lime juice. Hugh would often still be working when I came home, and of course I was even less motivated to work than when I'd left.

Several months passed in this pleasant manner, although it is possible my roommate's diligence was working insidiously on my conscience. To be formally admitted to the physiotherapy education programme, students studied the basic subjects for nine months and then took an entry examination. Those who passed then completed the first year and progressed to the second year. Those who failed repeated the nine months and re-sat. It suddenly became rather obvious to me that I would probably fail the entry stage unless I did some real work. With only three or four weeks before the examinations I realized that Bramwell knew everything about everything and more. Perhaps I also remembered Mr Mills from college – all his help and the wonderful chance I had been given. I gave it my all in those final weeks, passed the exam and was accepted into the next phase of the programme.

The physiotherapy curriculum at Dunedin was identical to programmes offered in the United Kingdom. Enid Gotz and Gwen Hislop, the principle instructors, had been recruited from Britain. The main elements were anatomy, biomechanics, therapeutic exercise and methods of applying electrical hocus-pocus gadgetry such as short-wave diathermy used to heat injured tissues, none of which involved the patient in his or her own recovery.

Miss Gotz, the Head of the Physiotherapy School at that time, was an outstanding figure. She was tall, with perfect posture and any student she caught slouching was in trouble. Sitting or standing slouched was an almost criminal offence in her eyes and the careless would be told in no uncertain terms that they were letting the whole school down! Her obsession with posture imprinted itself in my thinking and later I realized it was the most important thing I learned in my training.

As all 20-year-old students should, I learned much more than the subjects of my chosen field. Although now a somewhat more conscientious student, I nevertheless found my life full of colour and friends.

Parties were frequent and beer was an essential expense in a student's budget. Ma Blaney's on Broadway in town was a favourite drinking spot for many of us and, always stretching the boundaries, we found it more exciting going to the 'pub' after legal hours, including on Sundays. I am not sure if it really happened this way, but it seemed as though at official closing time the cops would phone and tell the barman they were on their way – checking the law was being obeyed. The barman, with not much more than a sweep of his arm, would erase all evidence of our presence from the bar top and order us all into the shed behind the pub. We knew the routine; we never argued, scrambling into the old woodshed and allowing the door to be padlocked behind us with a heavy chain. We remained there, silencing those who felt they had to sing, until the barman came and released us for many more hours of merriment inside. They were great days.

Of course we drank more that we should have. I recall making my way home on one of these Sundays feeling more than slightly unsteady on my feet. I decided a brief rest in a gloomy doorway would help me recover my bearings. I noticed a policeman making his way down the opposite side of the street dutifully checking with his torch to see if the doors of the shops were secure. Resisting the urge to flee and be judged guilty of something more sinister, I remained in the doorway hoping the officer would not notice me. Unfortunately I had unwittingly chosen a spot beside an empty methylated spirits bottle. As this 'evidence' was suddenly illuminated by the torch, I found myself explaining to the gendarme, I hoped convincingly, that the bottle and I were together by an unfortunate coincidence.

Whatever he thought about this he obviously decided I was unfit to make it home on my own. He called a taxi, muttering something about bloody students as he put me into it to be taken home. I had spent all my money that night so the officer paid the driver and told me to return the money to the police station. I very gratefully did so the next morning. Recalling my earlier contact with the police in Masterton over my stolen two pennies, this incident was yet further confirmation to me of the benevolence of our men in black.

Student days in Otago were wonderful in other ways too. There were five men and 45 women enrolled in Physiotherapy and we had nearly all come straight from secondary school. The women were eagerly courted by the numerous young medical students at the university – and clearly for most of them a young doctor would have had more potential as a husband than we did. Although we had serious competition, we never wanted for female company.

In the winters I played field hockey and was selected in 1952 to play for the university. I often played chess at the local club in the evenings, when undoubtedly I should have been going over our lectures. But of course we worked hard when we had to; our programme was demanding and exams had to be passed. I do remember being sceptical even then about some of the treatments that were recommended for joint and muscular aches and pains. The treatment options we were taught to administer included strengthening and mobility exercises, massage, infra-red heat, ultraviolet treatment for skin complaints, short-wave diathermy and various electrical stimulative procedures.

During the second year we had short-term placements. I was allocated the Dunedin Hospital chest ward, where it was the physiotherapist's responsibility to ensure the patient practiced deep-breathing exercises following surgery in an attempt to hasten the return to normal function. In the 1950s tuberculosis was still widespread and surgical removal of a lung or procedures to collapse the lung or lungs was common.

While I was on the chest ward a patient I was seeing died following such surgery. Her extensive wound became so infected that during the deep-breathing exercises it would open and close because strapping would not adhere to the surrounding suppurating flesh. After reporting this to the head nurse I was assured that this was not unusual in such cases and that they would deal with it later. I saw the patient each of the following few days but decided, despite being told to continue, I could not put her through what appeared to be an exercise in futility. I just talked to her and hoped she would get better. About the third day I went once more as instructed – the bed was empty, made up with clean sheets. This affected me deeply and almost immediately I decided that I could not work in situations where that could happen.

So the years passed. Tension was high while we waited for our results following our final examinations in October 1952. Finally they were posted on the wall of the social room at the school. Three of our group of five men passed and I was one of them, but our joy was marred by the failure of our two close friends. We had formed really strong bonds over three very full years together.

Shortly after this I received notice from the Army that my military training, compulsory at the time but suspended for university study, was now to be commenced. I thought this would be a terrible waste of my education. Here I was, qualified and ready to treat the waiting masses of patients' aches and pains and instead I would be playing at being a soldier for three months.

At the same time the Health Department issued orders for me to begin service at Silverstream Hospital, near Wellington; I was 'bonded' to the government for three years to repay my university education costs.

Just after my graduation and briefly back in Masterton, I was taken aback when my father asked to see me. He had never before initiated contact with me. Our meeting was a bit stiff at first as we were both guarded and I was very nervous. After a lengthy lunch with a few ales – and then a whiskey or two – I found my father to be a most entertaining character, full of stories of his life as a lawyer and his hobby, golf. I realized too, that this remote figure in my life was very proud of me – his son. I wished I had had more opportunities to meet him.

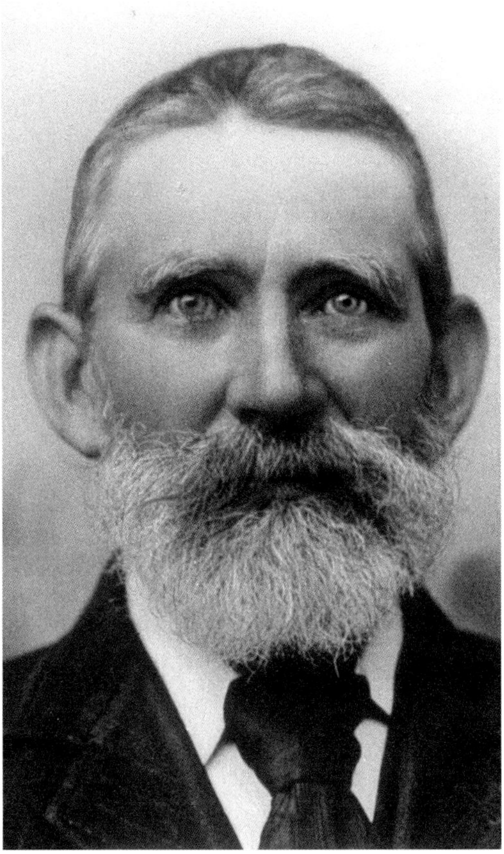

Grandfather Roderick McKenzie, c.1880.

Roderick's house at Fernridge near Masterton, c.1893. My father is sitting behind the dog.

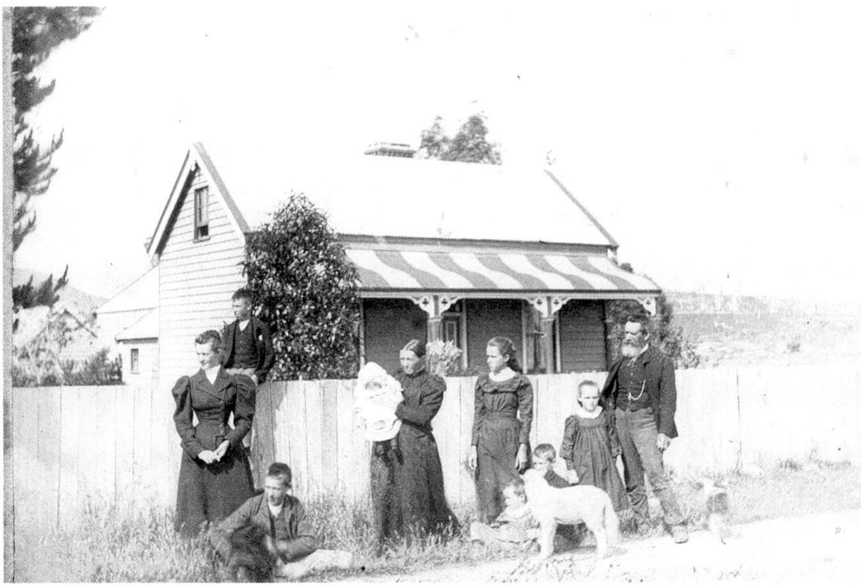

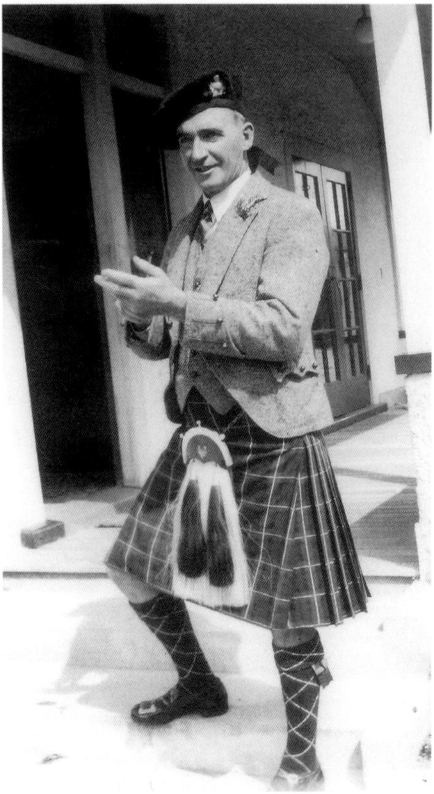

My father, Robert McKenzie, c. 1938.

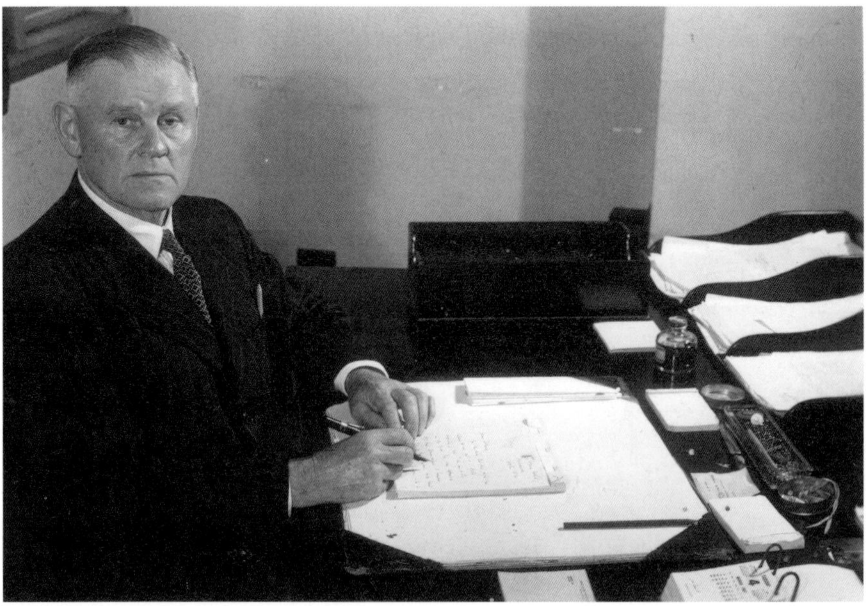

Jim Thorn, my uncle and member of the first Labour Government.

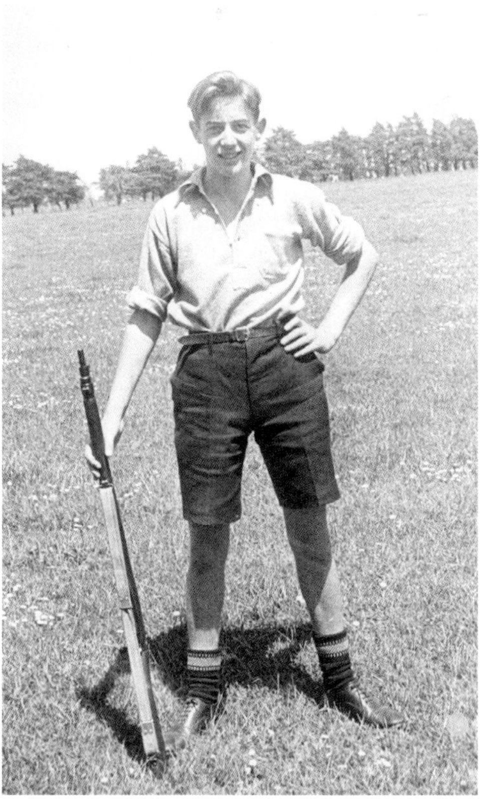

Wairarapa College rifle shooting champion 1948 and 1949.

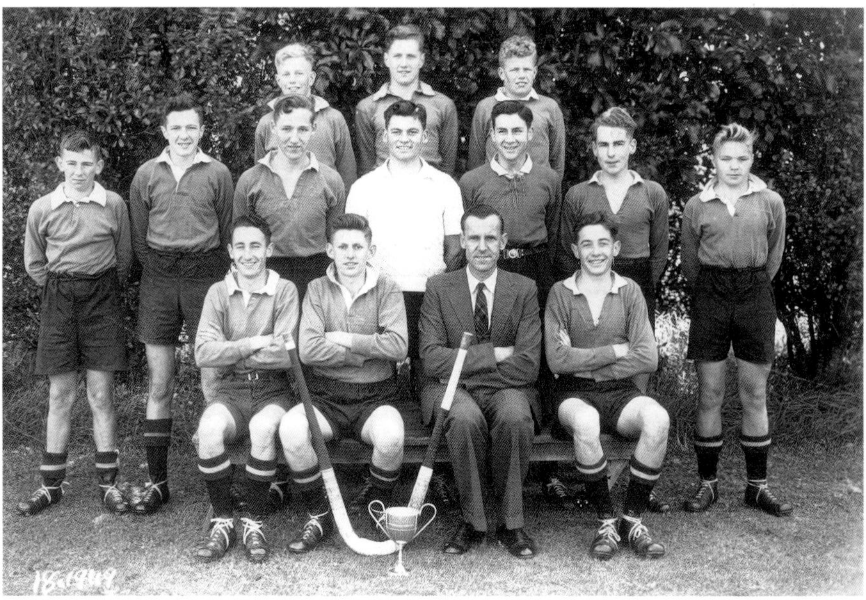

Wairarapa College hockey team 1948. I am on the right, seated.

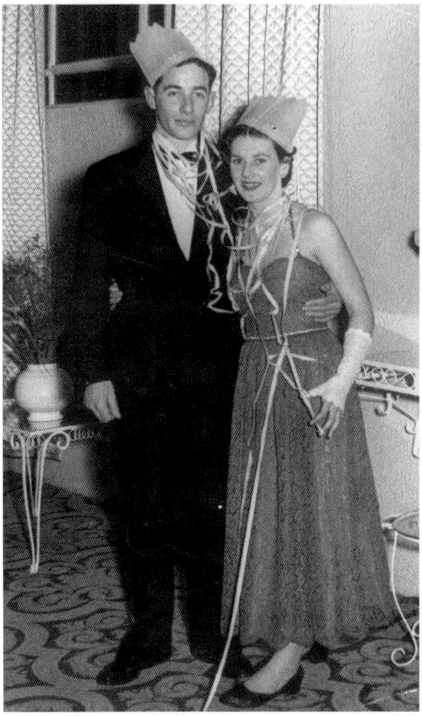

With Joy at the Majestic Cabaret, Wellington in 1954.

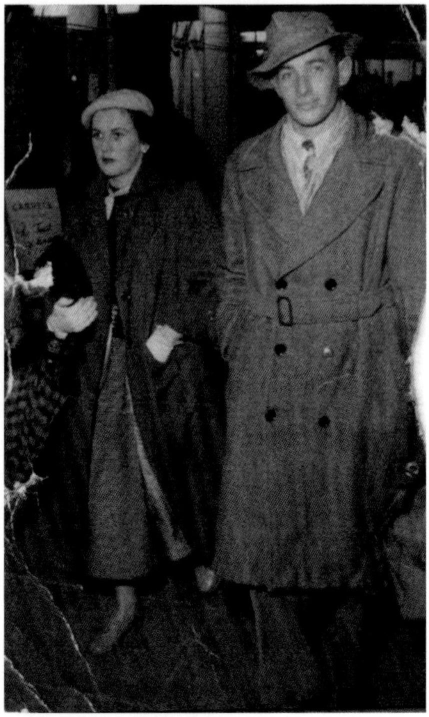

Mid-winter shopping.

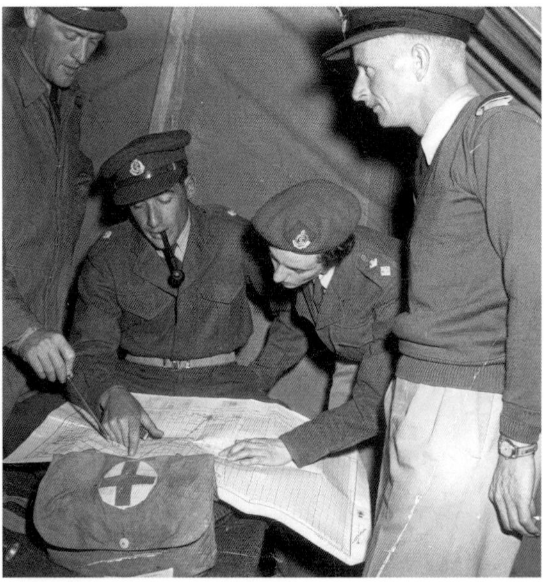

Briefing at 2nd General Hospital NZ Army Medical Corps camp, 1956. I'm the one with the pipe.

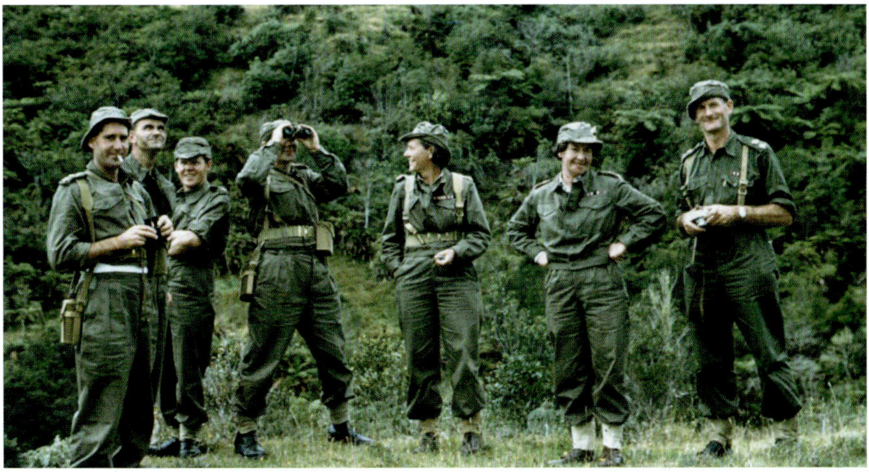

Officers of 2nd General Hospital on manoeuvres, 1956. I was the photographer.

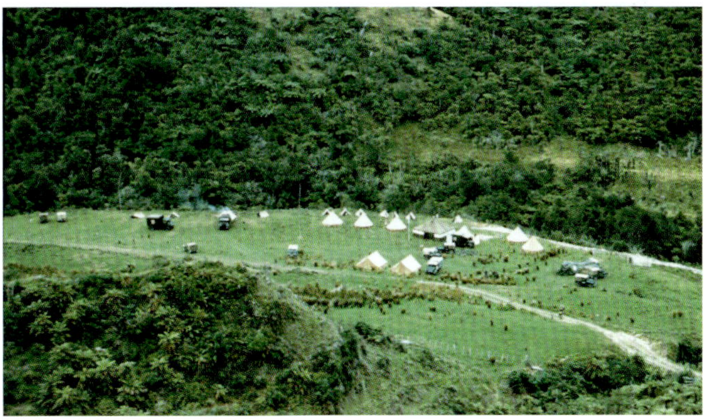

Setting up tented hospital, 1956.

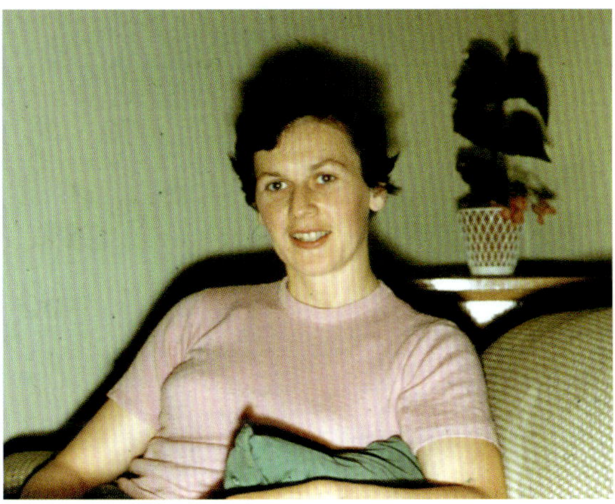

Joy in our flat, 1957.

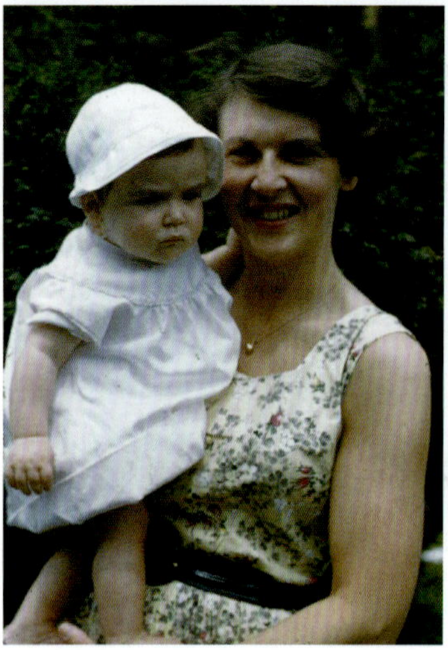

Joy and our daughter, Jan, 1959.

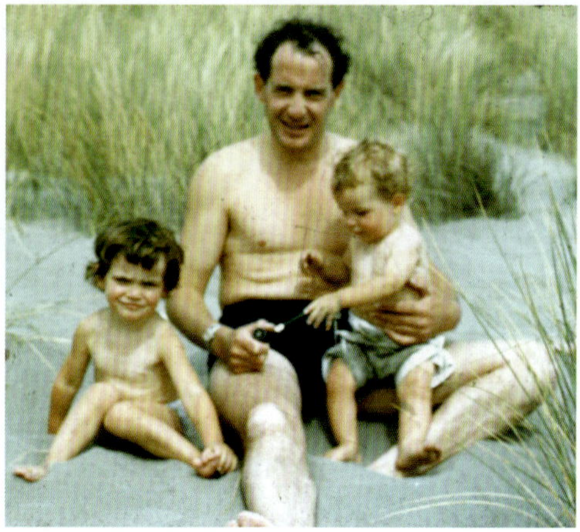

With Jan and son David.

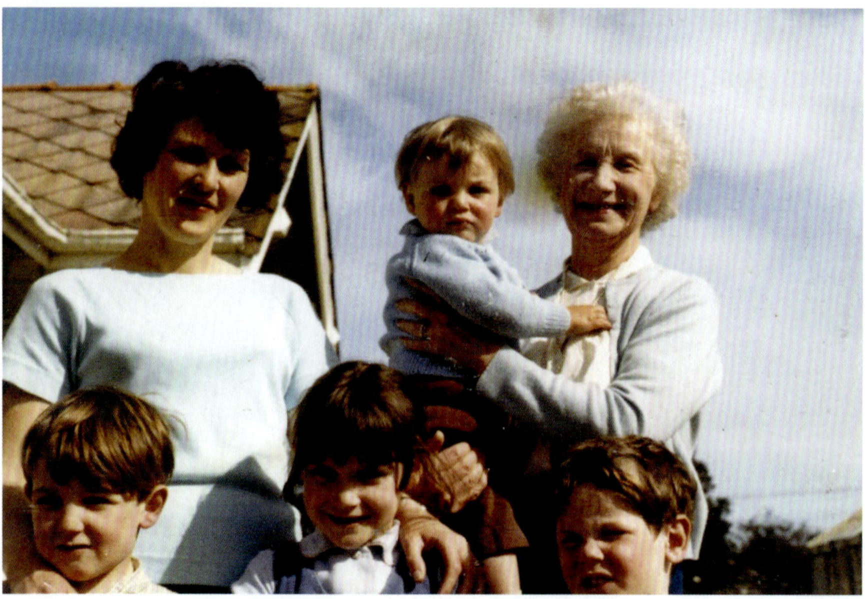

My mother with Joy and the children.

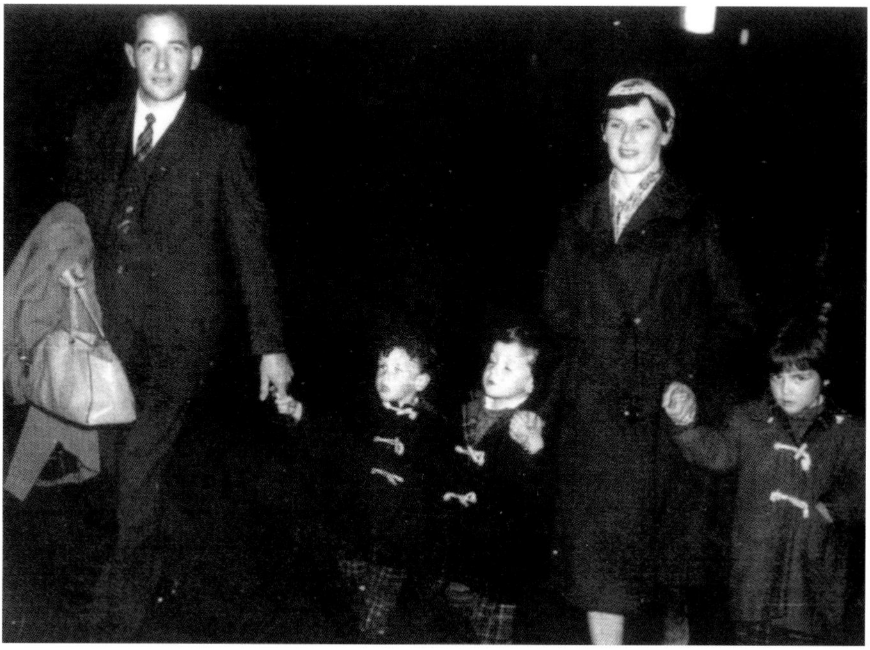

A small handful, 1962.

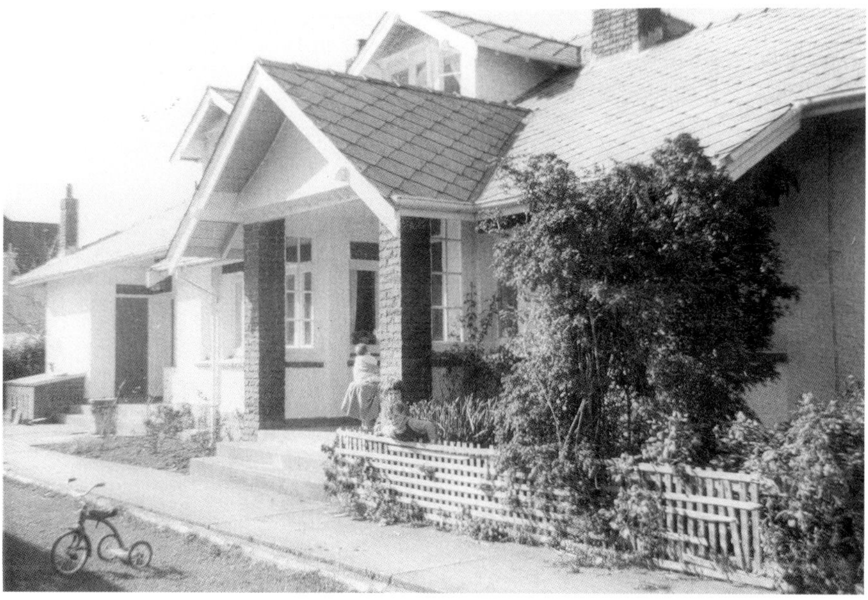

Our house in Cornwall Street, Lower Hutt, 1963.

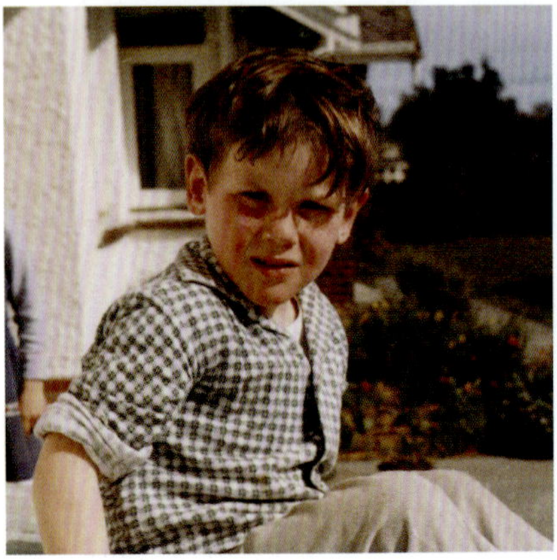

Alistair at Cornwall Street, 1965.

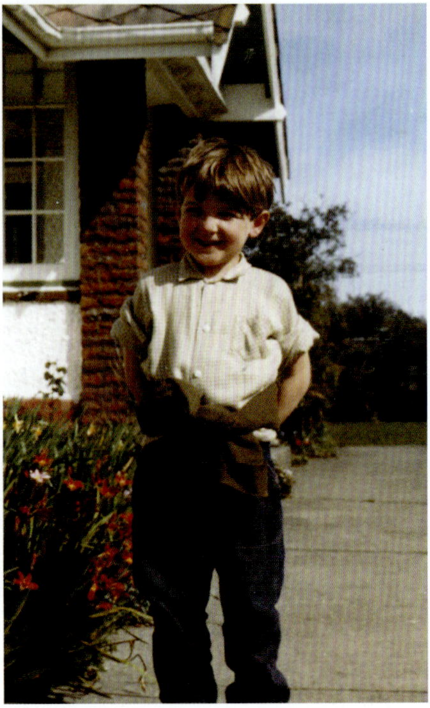

David at Cornwall Street, 1966.

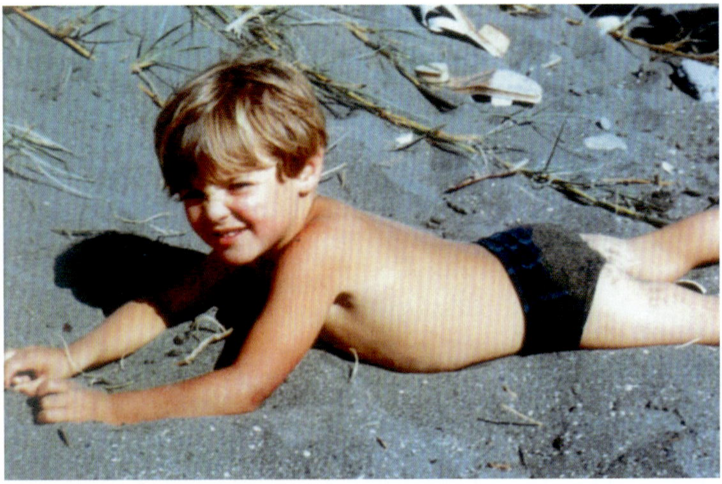

Andrew at the beach, 1967.

At this new turning point, I could only feel that life was good. I was more eager than ever for whatever lay ahead.

I was to commence working at Silverstream Hospital three weeks after graduation early in November. There was enough time to take a short summer holiday, and as I had seen very little of my own reputedly beautiful country I decided I would hitchhike around the North Island. I had hardly any money but Mum gave me £10 and I set forth with only a change of clothes and a sleeping bag.

I had many pickups – some just lasted a few miles, but many took me well along my way. I stayed in one small hotel for 15 shillings and another, rather filthy one, for ten shillings a night. I was often in awe of the wonderful scenery I was seeing for the first time and I also met some very interesting people.

After travelling up the centre of the island, over the Desert Road, past the volcanoes Mt Ruapehu and Mt Ngauruhoe, and Lake Taupo just to the north of them, I chose to head out to the East Coast. One of my lifts was on the back of a truck carrying long power poles and other equipment for their erection. I worked my way between the poles, hoping they were secure, and leaned against a stack of sacks for a long and bumpy ride. One of the sacks must have contained an oily black substance, as to my distress it left a large black stain on the back of my university blazer, the only jacket I had.

On reaching the small, isolated town of Taneatua, I called at the only store in sight – an old wooden building with a faded banner painted with the words 'The Great Taneatua General Store'. I felt I had been cast back 30 years in time when, after ringing the bell and waiting for several minutes, a very old man appeared wearing a long black apron, a white shirt and a tie. I asked him if he had any dry-cleaning fluid. He didn't think so. He called to someone out the back and I heard a female voice reply that they didn't because no one ever asked for it. So I asked if they had any carbon tetrachloride, which I thought would serve the same purpose. The man disappeared, reappearing after a while to report that his wife said that the firm that used to make it had gone out of business. My stain and I were clearly going to stay together and I decided to put it out of my mind.

Then I asked a Maori man sitting in his car outside how far it was to Gisborne through the Waioeka Gorge south of the town, and with his answer of 40 or 50 miles, I set forth and hoped that I would soon get a ride. I was a few miles into the gorge when I came across a car parked on the opposite side of the road. Steam was gushing from the front of the car as its driver poured water into the radiator. He asked me where I thought I was going, and when I said to Gisborne he muttered that if I was expecting a lift I would be disappointed as very few cars travelled on this road at night. He did, however, think that the Works truck would come through at one in the morning.

Should I go on in hope, or go back and find a place to stay in Taneatua, which, from what I had seen of the town, might also be difficult? I went on. By this time it was about 9:30 in the evening and there was just enough light to see the road. By 11:30 still no cars had passed in either direction. I put my pack in the centre of the road and got into my sleeping bag a little off the road. I woke to the throaty sound of an approaching engine and lept onto the road to join my pack. To my enormous relief the Works truck driver stopped. He was going to Gisborne but would be stopping in the middle of the gorge at the Works camp.

The road was very narrow, unpaved, and required constant maintenance. The men who did the maintenance worked in the gorge for three weeks and then had a week's break. This night was the end of their three-week shift and they were having the usual party. The truck driver was always invited and I had no option but to join in and hope that he would be sober enough afterwards to get us to Gisborne.

Soon a very large glow in the dark ahead indicated we were near the camp. A huge bonfire was raging. I will never forget that night, the party, and the Maori maintenance workers. There were no Pakeha (the Maori name for Europeans) apart from the truck driver and myself. Around the fire there appeared to be about an acre of cleared land, with some small wooden huts spread around the clearing.

I presumed the larger fire was for light, warmth and atmosphere as there was a smaller fire on which a pig or lamb was roasting. A tracked excavator lifted logs onto the bonfire whenever it showed any sign of dying back. There were two large kegs of beer from which the men were continuously filling jugs. These were passed around the 30 or so workers who would drink and pass to a mate. I could see it would be bad form if I did not get into the swing of it all and steeled myself to drink as they did as the jugs came past. It was already a very jolly occasion when we arrived – evidence of the effects of the good ale.

I too was enjoying it all very much. I remember one of the older Maori asking me what had brought me into the gorge in the middle of the night. I told him what I'd being doing and my plans for the future. He asked what I would be telling my friends about this night once back in Wellington. He wanted to know if I'd say I enjoyed a wonderful feast with some Maori friends, or that I'd met a whole lot of drunken black bastards. I pondered this and realized that there was considerable resentment among these isolated indigenous people for earlier colonial injustices that still had not been righted. Many years later I understood more fully the tensions in the Maori–Pakeha relationship and the effect on Maori tribal life of the land losses they had suffered. Compensation by the Government was still years away.

After we left the party my truck driver, who was now very late and possibly very drunk, drove at considerable speed to Gisborne. We parted company there and after I had had breakfast I continued my travels south through Hawke's Bay and eventually back down to Silverstream hospital. All in all it had been a very enjoyable break, but I was really now looking forward to working – and earning – for the first time.

CHAPTER 3

MILITARY SERVICE

I reported for duty at Silverstream Hospital at the end of November 1952. This prefabricated collection of buildings had been erected by the United States Marines to take in the sick and injured from the Pacific battles against the invading Japanese armies. It had not been intended for long-term use, but the Government Health Department decided it would continue to be used for long-term care patients. I was allocated a small apartment close to the main building and set about familiarizing myself with my surroundings and my patients. I could not help also noticing that there were some very attractive nurses at the hospital. One in particular had dark hair, blue eyes, and I thought she was just beautiful – Joy Johnston. Before I knew it I was in love. As we were both residents at the hospital compound, Joy and I would meet frequently. I started to resent my looming and inescapable military service even more.

Miss Pat Andrews, the charge physiotherapist at Wellington Hospital, was furious to learn that the newly minted colleague from Otago University would be interrupting employment at the satellite Silverstream Hospital for Army obligations. But the Army could not be argued with. At that time the policy required 14 weeks of compulsory military training for all New Zealand's young men. At age 18 we were conscripted into the Navy, Army or Air Force according to the nature and quality of our education. Those of us who went to university had our training postponed until we had completed our courses.

As expected, at the beginning of December I received word that I was to report for training at Linton Military Camp in late January

1953. The camp was just outside Palmerston North, some two hours' drive north of Wellington. Because of my university qualification I was drafted into the Royal New Zealand Army Medical Corps and attached to the 2nd General Hospital. This was in fact not a hospital of bricks and mortar, but a notional unit made up of tents and equipment in storage for the annual camps.

I duly completed the first four weeks of basic training at Linton Camp, and then we conscripts were allowed three days' leave before the next stage. I was desperate to get back to Wellington to see Joy, as the four weeks had seemed far too long to be apart. Our letters, while wonderful, were a poor substitute for being together.

The remaining ten weeks' training were to be completed at Waiouru Camp, located just south of Lake Taupo in the middle of the North Island, another two hours' drive north. Waiouru was a desolate, exposed outpost of civilization, almost entirely given over to the military camp and adjacent to the active volcano Mt Ruapehu at an altitude of 3,000 feet.

Freezing winds even in late summer made conditions extremely unpleasant as most of the training occurred in the surrounding exposed high desert country. Night temperatures were often below zero and minimal heating in the barracks meant there was much complaining, often in colourful and unrepeatable terms.

Although my mind was set against this untimely interruption in my life, I eventually came to see that this regimented training was one of the best things that could have happened to me. I had drifted through my schooling without much self-discipline, and without establishing a purpose or goals for my personal and professional betterment. Also I was not very physically fit. The Army gave me a huge boost in mental and physical confidence. Army discipline taught me self-discipline and I emerged heavier, stronger and more mentally focused, believing I could do anything I chose to do.

In Waiouru I was promoted to Corporal and was given the charge of a platoon. It was the only platoon in the Medical Corps that had a conscript in charge; all the others were under the command of professional, full-time non-commissioned officers. I had no idea at all of what was expected of me and as all in the platoon were also conscripts it was an enormous challenge for me to exercise my new-found authority. After a few weeks the platoon realized that perhaps they should let up on this amateur corporal, but, regardless, we remained the worst platoon in the brigade.

I had not sought leadership, and did not want it, instinctively knowing that to be given rank over my fellow conscripts was to guarantee their hostility. At the end of the training there was to be a passing-out parade in which the troops would march before the brigade commandant, the officers and the invited public. My platoon had been the worst in dress, drill and everything else through the first weeks of corps training. But perhaps they were tired of their lowly status, because an amazing thing happened to the men at the passing-out parade. When they marched through the parade ground the transformation was spectacular – they were voted the best platoon in the parade and were publicly complimented by the Commanding Officer. While I could hardly believe what had happened, I felt enormous pride in our achievement.

In the Military one was obliged to do things one normally would not do, and refusing to do them was not an option. Of course some of the 18-year-old conscripts had to learn things the hard way and a few even found themselves in Ardmore Military Prison for refusing to follow orders. They rarely offended a second time. On hearing their stories of confinement and punishment, I had no desire to step out of line in this environment. Later in civilian life, however, I learned that stepping out of line was sometimes the only way to resolve difficulties, and if you believed in what you were doing, you should see it through no matter what.

On the evening before our passing-out parade I was told I had been selected for a four-week officer-training course, to begin immediately. I knew that this further absence would be a real issue for Miss Andrews and I telephoned the hospital with some trepidation. She was not able to come to the phone and it was with a sense of relief that I decided to leave a message for her. Whether it was the further delay, or some other perceived failure in etiquette, when I eventually took up my position at Silverstream my relationship with this woman was rather difficult and unhappy.

With the extended officer training course completed, and having gained the rank of Second Lieutenant, I was posted to the local Territorial Army medical unit, the 2nd General Hospital. Thereafter, I was to undertake two weeks of further training each year. These annual duties were essentially occasions for bands of amateur soldiers to play at imaginary war. For some they provided a most enjoyable break from their regular occupations. Simulating injuries and treating them was a rather unrealistic part of our activities, but to our amusement, some of the troops – those with better imaginations – quite successfully feigned injury, disability and even paralysis. So convincing was one soldier's paralysis after a fall that he was almost on the way to the local hospital before suddenly miraculously recovering.

Sharing barracks with the boys on these training courses reminded me of my boarding school days and our ten-a-side dormitories. Over our weeks together, through our shared experiences both at work and at leisure, many durable friendships were formed. Warren Austad, a fellow conscript, is still one of my closest friends. We have shared many interests – sailing, golf, and at one time we developed an orchard together. Warren completed his medical training after the Army interruption and, following overseas experience, set up his practice in Wellington.

Another great friend from the Army days was Graeme Law. Graeme, Warren and I formed a lasting friendship and met with our wives at least once a year for dinner and to talk about the old times together in Her Majesty's Service. After our initial training Graeme joined the Territorial Army and pursued a degree in Law. In 1964 he became an officer in the Regular Army and was later made Director of Defence Legal Services, with the rank of Colonel.

There were many others I met and formed friendships with through the Army and our paths continued to cross throughout our professional lives. In my early days in practice in Wellington I was supported by Marshall Luke, a cardiologist, who frequently referred patients to me with back or neck problems; Ponty Hallwright, another cardiologist; Moore Tweed, a rheumatologist; and Evan Raine, a general surgeon. These relationships were invaluable, providing helpful introductions to the wider medical community in Wellington that were to last all my professional life.

But I am getting ahead of myself – I had yet to discharge my obligations to the Government, and now returned to work.

CHAPTER 4

EARLY DAYS IN PRACTICE AND MARRIAGE

At Wellington Hospital I was met by a very angry Miss Andrews, who demanded an explanation for my extended absence. My justification that I had no choice but to comply with the Army's requirements seemed to fall on deaf ears – or at least unsympathetic ones.

I would now begin what was intended to be a three-year tenure in hospital service. Silverstream cared for patients who had cerebral palsy, strokes and other neurological and long-term orthopaedic conditions. There was little in those days that could be done to help most of these patients and the therapists were charged with keeping them moving to whatever extent was feasible. Some of the post-surgical orthopaedic patients who were there to recover their mobility were exceptions. However, their recovery too was very slow, with little improvement being visible from one week to another.

I remember feeling great frustration that I could do so little for these people and it reduced my enthusiasm for the three years ahead of me. I had the impatience of youth and wanted to see rapid improvements from treatment. Worse still was that not a week passed without someone dying, usually from respiratory complications or heart disease. The only consolation was that here at Silverstream I was close to Joy.

I joined the Wellington branch of the New Zealand Society of Physiotherapists at this time. We were a small group, just six members. One day a fellow member, Keith Ritson, phoned to tell me that another physiotherapist in the city, 70-year-old Adeline O'Connor, had suffered a heart attack and would not be able to continue with her clinic. He wondered if I might be able to look after her regular patients. Miss O'Connor had commenced practice in 1919, when veterans were returning from the First World War. Many had severe injuries and they were treated variously with massage, electrotherapy and exercise.

Keith's proposal excited me although I was somewhat surprised that he considered me suitable to fill the role. But realism prevailed and I explained to him that I could not take up the offer due to my bond position. Shortly after this I was sharing my disappointment with a pleasant and chatty patient, telling her how much I would have liked to have accepted the offer. She had had her hip replaced with the one of the first metal implants that had become available and I was working with her to help her recover movement. Out of the blue she volunteered to lend me the money to pay off my bursary, which would free me from the obligation to continue working at the hospital. Paying off my bursary had not even seemed a remote possibility, but now the idea, with this totally unexpected generosity, was irresistible. So at age 23, with just the hospital experience of the past six months behind me, I began work in my own clinic on 7 December 1953 at 64 The Terrace in Wellington. Being the anniversary of the attack on Pearl Harbour, I wondered whether this was a good or bad omen.

Adeline O'Connor's rooms contained a large array of old electrotherapy equipment that had been in common use in the early part of the 20th century. None of us knew how to use these devices and they seemed fascinatingly grotesque. One gave off a spectacular shower of sparks when placed near the body, another apparently caused severe and painful muscular contractions, and yet another device decompressed the skin and muscle over which it was placed and would leave redness and bruising for several days. I read later that this was all to do with something called 'counter irritation'. I never did understand the purpose or efficacy of any of these machines, and, as none had ever been demonstrated to us at the Physiotherapy School, I had no intention of using them. I sent them to Dunbar Sloanes, the auctioneers who guaranteed to sell any object presented. In this promise they failed, for Miss O'Connor's electrotherapy instruments there were no buyers. Today they would probably be rare and priceless objects.

In my first week in practice I saw ten patients, but the next week this number doubled and continued to increase until I was seeing up to 40 patients a day in my very cramped premises. About a year later another physiotherapy practice was advertised for sale in a building not far away on the same street, in Kelvin Chambers. This space would easily accommodate the numbers of patients I was now seeing and furthermore I could now afford to purchase it. I did so. My career now seemed to be progressing very well. The demand for physiotherapy in the city was high and there were only seven practitioners there at the time. There was my mentor Keith Ritson and the rest were women, mostly practicing part time. I visited all of the doctors in the area and requested their support. This was considered the courteous thing to do at the time – it was marketing really. The doctors were quite supportive, especially the general practitioners, and I was soon working 10 or 11-hour days to keep up with the referrals that came to me.

Kelvin Chambers, located at 16 The Terrace, was in the centre of the business section of Wellington and also near Parliament and many government offices. Consequently my patients were often civil servants, business and professional workers and I rarely had an unpaid bill. My practice's location had me treating many officials in the Government, including Ministers of the Crown and successive Prime Ministers, Sir Sidney Holland, Sir Keith Holyoake, Sir Jack Marshall, Sir Robert Muldoon and David Lange.

Shortly after taking on Miss O'Connor's clinic, I was asked to call at the residence of Prime Minister Sir Sidney Holland, who had a severe pain in his lower back. Sir Sydney was lying on his back in bed in considerable discomfort. I was asked to give him heat treatment and massage but it was clear that this would not be possible as he was unable to turn to lie face down. I tried to help him to stand up, but once on his feet he immediately collapsed to the floor, crying out in agony. I had never before seen a patient in such pain. What had I done? Was he paralyzed? I could see the headlines in the morning paper: 'Prime Minister Sydney Holland seriously injured by incompetent novice therapist.' Thankfully, he gradually improved over the next few days and did not hold me in any way responsible.

The most entertaining of these notables was Prime Minister Keith Holyoake; he had a wonderful sense of humor. For a while I spent some 30 or 40 minutes every second day with Sir Keith and during these sessions he entertained me with what seemed an endless repertoire of amusing anecdotes from his long tenure in office. He also offered me some very good advice. I had been pondering whether or not to purchase a property priced well beyond our means and must have seemed distracted. He asked me what was on my mind and when I told him, his unequivocal advice was, "Buy it now, it will never be cheaper!" I could not afford to follow his advice at that time but I always remembered this dictum from our nation's leader and never again hesitated over such decisions.

At the same time all of this was happening I was courting Joy, with whom I was very much in love. During my short stint at Silverstream Hospital, where we had spent many hours together, I had unfortunately been caught by the caretaker helping Joy through the nurses' dorm window at 2 a.m., long after curfew. Joy had immediately been transferred to Hutt Hospital by the imperious and incensed Matron. Clearly I was watched over by an ever-present guardian angel as shortly afterwards I was to leave as well and take up practice in Wellington.

I must share a third encounter I had with the Police, in 1953 while courting Joy. I had been to visit her at the Hutt Hospital and was returning to Silverstream Hospital. It was about 1:30 a.m. – late enough that the buses and trains were no longer running, and far enough out of the way that no taxis were about. I was trying to hitchhike home on the Hutt Road. There were very few vehicles on the road at this hour, but finally one approached and stopped. Out popped two policemen to inquire what I was doing. When they were satisfied that I was not drunk, one told me to get off the side of the road. I objected that I could not be seen by passing motorists from the walking path, but I was again told to get off the roadway. My next objection – I thought under my breath – included among other choice items, the term "Gestapo". I was then summarily thrown headfirst into the back of the car and taken to the police station. During the questioning there, the night sergeant became very upset when after he asked me to spell "physiotherapist", I rattled off the spelling too quickly for him to keep up. After three attempts, he gave up. I was not charged and was told to go home. Now I objected that they had taken me miles out of my way and lost me a good deal of time as well. The sergeant dismissed me in exasperation and I again began the journey home. After I had been walking for some considerable time a car approached and, to my relief, stopped. It was the original policemen, who then offered me a ride to Silverstream Hospital, joking that at some point they might be in need of my professional services.

Joy and I were married on 23 September 1954. We had a very small wedding in Karehana Bay, Plimmerton, attended by Joy's parents, my mother, Joy's sister, Mina, and her husband, Rennick. I was truly overjoyed to be marrying the love of my life, but the occasion and the time thereafter was marred by my mother's disapproval and resentment of Joy. I could only conclude that she was jealous and did not want to share her son with anyone else.

After Joy and I were married we rented a one-bedroom flat on The Terrace just half a mile south of Kelvin Chambers. Joy was working as a nurse in a medical practice close by so we were both busy during the working week. We didn't have a garden, and little was required to clean and tidy the flat. These were hectic but very happy days.

One night, just a few weeks after we were married, in the early hours of the morning I woke and became aware of faint noises at the back of the house in the vicinity of the bathroom. Certain that we had a burglar inside the flat I very quietly got out of bed, careful not to wake Joy. I still had a 303 rifle from earlier hunting days in the Wairarapa and I quietly loaded it. I moved to the kitchen door and in the light of my torch saw the handle of the door start to turn.

I immediately turned the torch off and as soon as the door was wide enough I thrust the rifle barrel against the intruder's stomach shouting "Stop right there!".

"It's me!", came Joy's terrified voice out of the dark.

Needless to say it took us quite a while to get back to sleep, and the experience bothered me for some time as I contemplated what might have been had I pulled the trigger.

Our combined incomes soon allowed us to seek better accommodation. We found an ideal two-bedroom apartment in a more modern building and continued to be very happy with our lot.

My practice grew quickly and I worked long hours. If a patient was not able to get out of bed due to back pain, I would call in at home after finishing at the clinic, a service that was much appreciated by the patients and their doctors and resulted in even more referrals.

My friend and colleague Keith Ritson had been in the Air Force during the war and following his discharge had established a thriving practice, with his services much sought after. We would get together whenever possible and talk endlessly about patients, treatment methods, new ideas and what was right – and wrong – with the Physiotherapy Society. Keith had been elected President of the New Zealand Society of Physiotherapists in the late 1950s and he introduced significant changes to the Society's direction and established policies on various issues confronting the profession. He and I agreed that the public perception of physiotherapists needed to be changed. Most therapists were in public hospital service and consequently, the Society's policies were focused only on their interests. With Keith's input, conditions for therapists in private practice improved; he had direct access to the Minister of Health and was able to negotiate improved remuneration from the Government's contribution to fees. As a result of his enormous efforts to give those in the private sector a voice, the Society appointed him the private practitioners' representative in negotiations with the Government. Keith influenced me in many ways and I learned a great deal from him about professional politics outside the daily routine of practice.

On an ordinary day in 1956, in my third year in practice, a gentleman with low back pain and symptoms radiating into the back of his right leg was referred to me for treatment. The patient's name is lost to memory, but I've called him Mr Smith. Mr Smith had been experiencing pain for three weeks. I treated him for a further three weeks but his condition remained the same. I was providing the recommended treatment regimen for low back pain, which at that time consisted of short-wave diathermy, massage and strengthening exercises. I was running a little behind schedule with my appointments, and seeing Mr Smith arrive in the waiting area I told him to go into the vacant treatment room and lie face down on the treatment table.

It was five to ten minutes before I could attend to this gentleman and when I saw him in this hyper-extended position I was alarmed. Mr Smith, an obedient fellow, was lying face down on the table as instructed. I had forgotten that room had just been used to treat a patient with a knee problem and the table had been left with the head-end raised so the patient could receive treatment sitting with the legs outstretched. This positioned Mr Smith with his head elevated and his back arched into an extreme position called 'extension'. The wisdom of the day was that patients with low back pain, and especially those with referred symptoms radiating into the buttock and leg, were to be treated with 'flexion' (bending forward and thus the opposite of extension)-based exercises and positions, and passive treatments such as short-wave diathermy or ultrasound. In fact, some practitioners warned that severe and permanent harm could be done to these patients by extending their backs. Trying not to show my concern, I informed Mr Smith that he had been in that position long enough and asked how he was feeling. To my surprise he enthusiastically replied that this was the best he had felt in over three weeks. I asked in what way he felt better and he responded that though his low back pain had increased, the pain in his leg was gone. Unsure as to the cause of the change in his symptoms, and assuming it would return, I got him off the table. The leg pain had gone. I told Mr Smith that that was sufficient treatment for that day but asked him to return the following day. He did and excitedly reported that his back pain was reduced and he had no leg pain. Puzzled, I decided that I would try the same position again – amazingly, he now felt no back pain at all.

This outcome was completely contrary to my expectations. There was no aggravation to his condition from the adoption of the extended position. Mr Smith was of course delighted; for the first time in six weeks he was free of pain – he was cured. I had little idea at the time that this patient and his treatment would shape the rest of my career and my life.

On 28 May 1957 our daughter, Jan, was born. I was very glad that my father, who had had a severe stroke just after Joy and I married, lived just long enough to see his first grandchild. We continued to live in the apartment but began now looking for a suitable house or land on which to build. After a year-long search we found a section and in a close-by Wellington suburb built our first family home.

CHAPTER 5

MR SMITH AND BUILDING THE THEORY

My experience with Mr Smith aroused both wonder and serious doubt in me. I began considering the possibility that the accepted treatment of back problems might be inappropriate in many situations. I found myself questioning everything I had been taught. I began to be particularly suspicious of the claims that were made regarding the value of electrical techniques. Having already read about the many possible causes of back problems, I found it difficult to imagine heat or cold or electricity altering dislocated or worn joints or disc tissue.

Mr Smith, in a position contrary to all established recommendations, recovered normal mobility and was pain free in a matter of 48 hours. According to accepted opinion of the day his condition should have worsened. The extreme extension position in which he was placed was considered a most inappropriate one, especially for a patient with sciatica. Serious compression of the sciatic nerve was thought certain to follow. This simply did not happen. So dramatic was this man's improvement that I had to contemplate the possibility that the theory around diagnosis and treatment of back problems might be wrong. While struggling to comprehend the reasons for Mr Smith's recovery, I naturally began to wonder if other patients would respond in this manner.

For the next year or so I placed every patient with low back pain and low back pain with sciatica and radiating symptoms in the extreme extension position, face down on that same table for five to ten minutes. I wanted to understand how Mr Smith's amazing recovery had occurred and as his relief had been rapid and caused no harm, cautious experimentation with others seemed important. I would question them continuously to determine if their symptoms were changing; their different responses often added to my confusion. I soon noted that if the position was helpful, they would report within a few minutes that the pain was diminishing.

The majority of patients responded rapidly in a similar manner to Mr Smith, but some did not. A few experienced increased pain that would sometimes spread and move down the leg, still others would slowly respond over several weeks, and some would not be affected in any way by the extreme position. Thus I had rapid responders, slow responders, non-responders and those whose condition was worsened.

Suddenly I had more questions than answers. What changes were occurring inside the spinal joints? Was healing at this speed possible? That seemed extremely unlikely because healing occurs over several weeks, not a day or two and certainly not within minutes. Was some tissue loose and free to move, thus allowing pain to move from one place to another? It seemed a more likely explanation. Why were patients' responses so varied? Why would pain sometimes move from one side of the back to the other? What caused pain to shift from the back to the leg? Why on some days did the pain affect the right leg and a few days later the left? Why were some patients totally pain free one day with sudden recurrence the next? These were just the first of many questions that came up.

Pondering all this, my first inspiration came from the work of Dr James Cyriax. I had been aware of the work of Cyriax, an orthopaedic physician at Wimpole Street, London, and had read his books on manipulation treatment for back problems. He attributed common back problems to injury or tearing of the disc lying between the vertebrae. The disc has a soft, gel-like inside and this can bulge in different directions when compressed. If the disc bulged sufficiently it would cause back pain, and if it was displaced it could cause sciatica as well. Did the rapid changes I was seeing result from a change in the volume and direction of displacement?

Dr Cyriax provided a very rational and plausible explanation for the cause of most back disorders and I was able to incorporate his thinking into my growing data on patients with back problems. The main difficulty was that there did not appear to be any other medical authority who believed Cyriax was right. I was to bear the burden of my belief in Cyriax for many years to come.

I became convinced that the disc could move between the joints from the pressure applied when the back was flexed or extended. When patients improved quickly, was the displaced disc being squeezed back into place? And when there was no change, was the disc fixed and unable to move, and if so why? Much later I observed from records that those who did not change rapidly had had their problem for many months, sometimes as long as six months to a year. What could cause the delay in response? Was it scarring as result of tissue healing? Cyriax believed that as all back pain came from the intervertebral disc, sudden pain must come from the outer part of it. If pain came on slowly, it must come from the gradual displacement of the soft inner part of the disc, the nucleus pulposus.

At this juncture I felt certain that Mr Smith's pain disappeared because the extreme extension of his back had changed the pressure on a displaced nucleus pulposus. Did that extension pressure reduce a bulging disc that in turn decreased the pressure on the adjacent nerve root which formed part of the sciatic nerve? Did a particular position make it possible to reverse disc displacement? That prospect was exciting indeed. What was to become known as the 'disc model theory' was evolving.

Now, about five years into practice, I had many patients and very full days and with only one treatment table with an adjustable end, I was under considerable time pressure. One day a new patient appeared who seemed likely to benefit from the sustained extension treatment, but with the table already occupied I had him lie on a flat table face down and asked him to place his hands under his shoulders and to push up, keeping his hips and legs flat on the table. I asked him to hold the extended position for as long as he could and then to lower himself to horizontal again. This replicated the position adopted by Mr Smith but was achieved by the patient relying solely on his own arm power. The only disadvantage was that the patient could not stay in that position for as long because of the effort involved.

That first patient reported that his pain was improved when his upper body was raised but it returned when he went down. I asked him to keep repeating the exercise and with each repetition he reported less pain. Over time I slowly realised that patients repeating the exercise themselves achieved the same, and in many cases superior, benefit to those lying on the table with the raised end. I was now convinced more than ever that long, slow pressure squeezed the disc and changed the internal distribution of fluids. This in turn reduced the symptoms. It explained the rapid and permanent relief many experienced from this treatment. The seed of patient self-treatment had been sown. I called this, simply, the 'push-up' exercise.

At that time I made another significant chance discovery. It concerned two patients I had recently seen who seemingly had identical pain and identical movement restrictions. Both had increased pain in the leg in bending forward, and it was worse with sitting, especially when driving. One was markedly better after only a few days of treatment, but the other was completely unchanged. How could such a different result be explained?

In those days I was recording all my patients symptom responses to movements albeit in a rudimentary fashion. I believe I was the first to record such responses and over time I began to understand how important these were. I became very diligent and detailed the many variations that occurred from patient to patient. The detail eventually allowed me to identify the three most common disorders found to affect all human musculoskeletal structures.

I re-examined the responses recorded previously on their assessment sheets. In the one case the patient had described his pain as gradually moving from the leg to the middle of his back as he exercised, during which time he recovered movement. He could then move further and further until he became pain free, and was then able to bend forward without experiencing the pain in his leg. Most of this occurred in just one treatment session. He had developed his symptoms only ten days previously. The patient whose symptoms were unchanged was able to bend forward and reach with his fingertips only to the knees and no further. No matter how often he repeated the extension movements his leg pain remained as before and became worse the further he bent. He described the pain as though a tight cord at the back of his leg were preventing the movement. He had had this problem for over six months. This example seemed to point to a connection between the length of time a patient had been suffering and the speed of recovery. And so, with the passage of time I was able to confirm the proposition.

I was reading every article about back problems in the medical journals available in New Zealand. I knew something about the findings of researchers who were operating on patients with severe back pain and sciatica. A research paper written in New Zealand in 1948 caught my attention. Neurosurgeons at Dunedin Hospital reported their findings from surgery on over 300 patients suffering from severe back pain or sciatica. Falconer, Begg and McGeorge found that the disc was a common cause of severe back pain and was the main cause of sciatica. They found that when many disc injuries healed, scar tissue tied itself to the nerve. This caused pain in the leg whenever the patient moved past a certain point and severely restricted forward bending movement.

Thus the unchanged patient of my duo could possibly have scarring bound to the nerve. That would account for the pattern of his pain and his restricted movement. Healing was brought about by scar-tissue formation, and it was well established that scar tissue tended to contract. Was this why some people with back pain responded slowly over weeks as repair progressed but remained stiff in the back, with limited movement? During forward bending, at a certain point the scar would be stretched and cause pain. Although healing was complete, they still felt pain in the original area as the scar tissue objected to the stretching. Patients would thus feel they were still suffering from the original injury and would avoid repeating the very movement that, if controlled well, would lead to recovery.

Slowly the pieces were coming together. Tissue from the disc could be displaced. 'Internal derangement syndrome' seemed a very satisfactory diagnosis. I could now identify the difference between the two most common causes of recurrent and persistent back pain simply by observing the behaviour of the pain in response to repeated exercise and without the need for X-rays. (CT and MRI scanners were yet to be invented.) Those who had evidence of scar tissue needed different management from those who had 'derangement syndrome'. But scars can be stretched and tissue remodelled with persistent and consistent exercise. It could take weeks instead of days, but once the problem was recognized the patient could be exercised or even be taught how to remodel his own contracted scar tissue.

'Dysfunction syndrome' seemed to be an appropriate umbrella name for these problems. The more I learned about the influence of movement on pain, the more I believed the disc model theory to be valid. Strain and eventual displacement of the disc, or scarring and repair of the injured disc, could explain the majority of common lower-back and neck problems.

However, it did not explain all spine problems. Some symptoms still defied my theories. Among the variations in the conditions I was encountering almost daily a very small proportion of patients complained of only occasional pain. When I asked them to go through my routine exercises, they consistently reported that none of these brought on their pain.

One such patient had no pain during his first examination. I had asked him to come back a few days later and in the meantime to note the circumstances causing any of his symptoms to appear. When he returned he waited seated for about 20 minutes. As he rose from the chair he exclaimed that he had pain on getting up to the standing position. I assumed he would experience pain during the examination, but he did not. On a previous occasion I had been a little behind schedule and two patients were sitting in the waiting room for longer than usual and both complained that the chairs were causing them more pain. The chairs in my waiting room were an old style, offering no support for the lower back (quite an indictment for a physio dedicated to treating the spine!). I wondered if this man's pain would reappear if he went back to the waiting room chair for another 20 minutes. After just a few minutes in the chair he said he could again feel the beginnings of the pain in the centre of his back. It seemed that the posture that sitting on the chair encouraged was slouched, with the lower back in a flexed position.

I now realized that both the pain caused by prolonged or repeated bending forward and the pain caused merely by sitting in a slouched position were caused by prolonged flexion in the lower back. Both situations may lead to internal derangement of the spinal disc.

If sitting slouched for prolonged periods could by itself lead to distortion and displacement of the lower spinal discs, I realized that preventing poor sitting posture was essential in the treatment of lower back pain. To correct and prevent the habit of slouched sitting amongst my patients I designed a lumbar roll which, when placed between the low back and the chair, prevented the adoption of poor posture.

As no such device of the appropriate dimensions was available commercially, Joy and I started making our own. Initially we made the covers from stretch vinyl and stuffed them with sheep's wool gathered from our small flock at End Farm. The numbers I required at the clinic in Kelvin Chambers grew to the extent that we decided to have them made professionally, and eventually these supports were marketed by the NZ Back Foundation to provide funds for research and education in Mechanical Diagnosis and Therapy (more on this later).

Now there were more questions. My slouching patient could not be experiencing a derangement of the disc, because he could move fully in all directions without pain. But why could I not bring on pain with exercise? Was this a problem with the disc, or simply caused by overstretching the ligaments supporting the disc and smaller joints of the spine? Did such patients have the beginnings of lower-back derangement or disc prolapse? Another chance observation helped me. One day when two of my sons were skylarking together, one put a hammer lock on the other and held it, causing yelps of pain from his victim. No harm had ever lasted from these antics commonly employed by the boys. It suddenly seemed obvious that pain comes on whenever even normal joints are over-stretched, but if no damage occurs it passes. This had to be the explanation for those patients who only have pain after prolonged unusual positioning. We should simply correct the position of the back. The dictum became: Do not sit slouched or remain in any extreme position – it's bad for your back! To help patients understand this most simple cause of pain, I used to hold one of their fingers bent back far enough to cause mild pain. On releasing the finger the pain would immediately disappear. Very few failed to understand that explanation.

I now described patients with these problems as having 'postural syndrome'. I designed back supports to aid correction of the sitting posture. Without adequate support, many who sit for any length of time tire and slump. Derangements may be corrected by the exercises, but successful correction is short-lived and will recur if the patient again sits slouched in flexion. This explained why some patients would feel fine after completing their exercises but found the pain reappeared after sitting relaxed in the car or an easy chair. I now kept a record of my patients' sitting habits – and their consequences. I found that a substantial majority of those with low back pain felt worse after prolonged sitting. The longer they remained sitting, the more likely it was that they would allow the lower back to flex.

I was dining in a large restaurant one evening about this time and observed that, almost without exception, the customers were relaxed – and slouched. At every opportunity thereafter I took notice of the postures that people adopted after they had been sitting for a while. The slouched sitting posture of humans in a relaxed context is almost universal – and so is potential back pain.

One thing led to another and the theory broadened. With the passing of time and the data from many hundreds of patients I began to see that lower back pain is caused by a cascade of events that are probably inevitable unless educational interventions are successful. At the beginning of the cycle patients get slight back pain after prolonged sitting, usually in a slouched, flexed position. There is no damage yet. The pain experienced on rising ceases after moving about. As it never lasts for long, the individual never worries

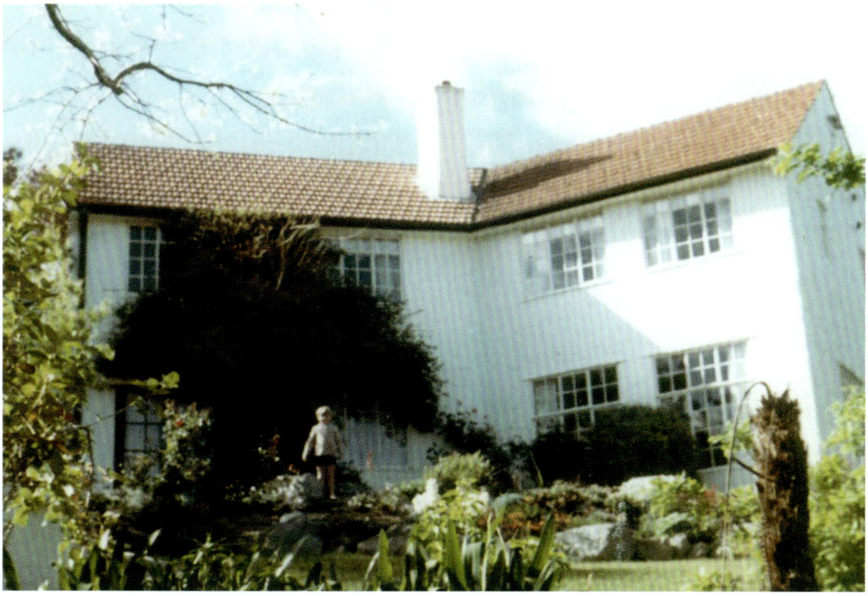

"Woodhill", our house in Silverstream, not far from the old hospital, where I first worked.

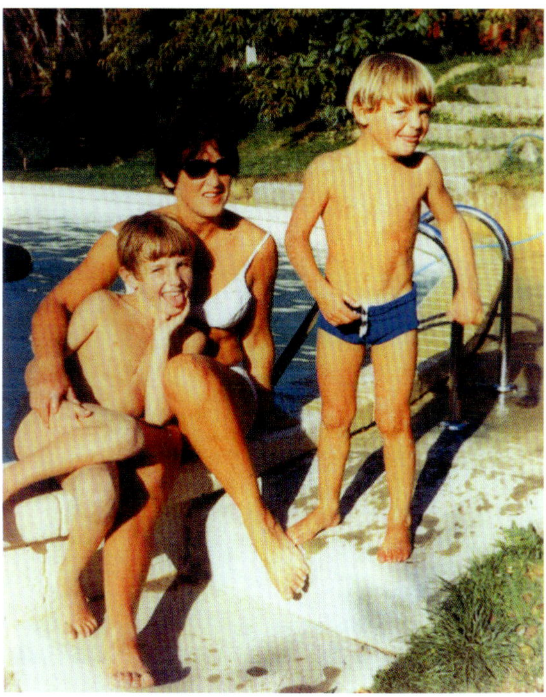

Joy with David and Andrew (standing) at "Woodhill".

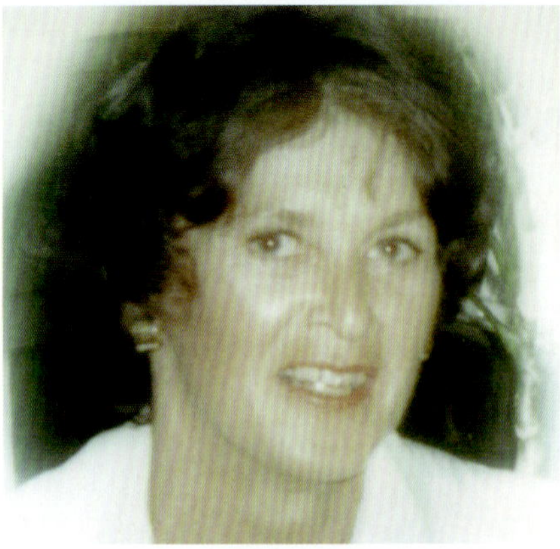
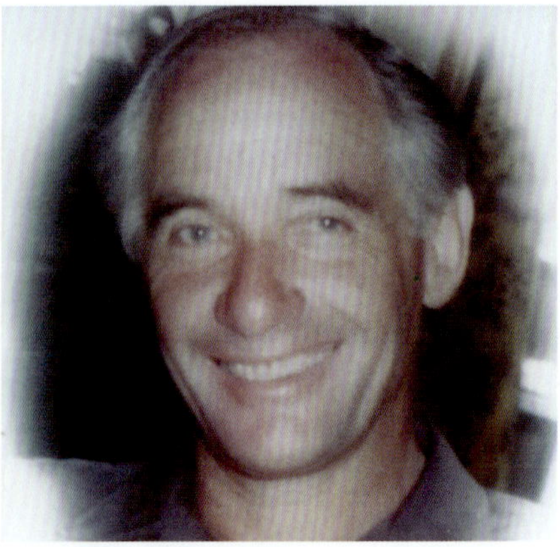

Joy and I in 1975.

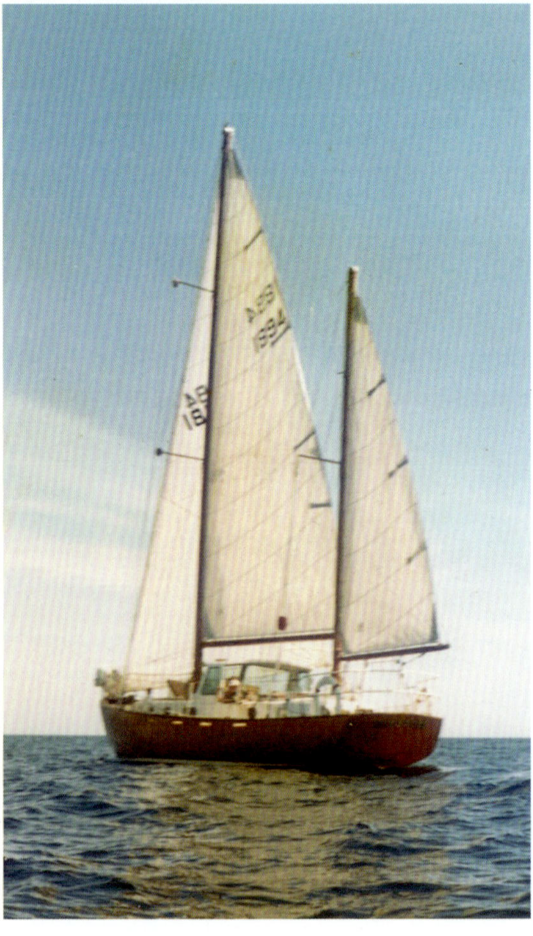

Our first yacht, Sundance, *at sea, early 1970s.*

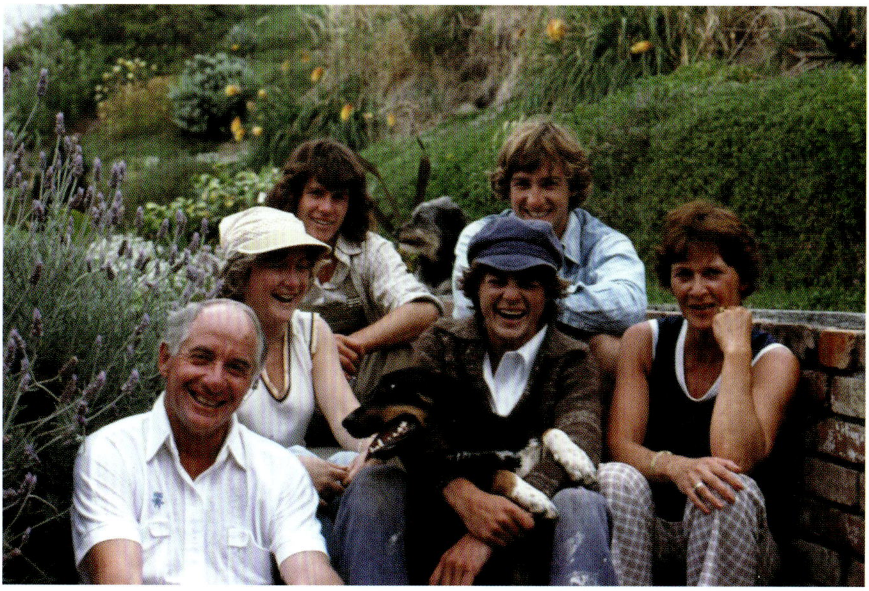

The whole family at End Farm, about 1980.

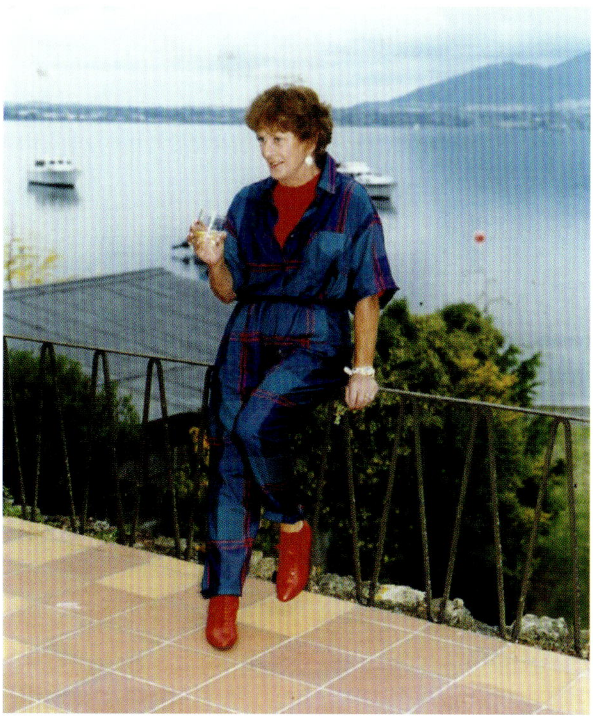

Joy at our cottage in the Marlborough Sounds, 1998.

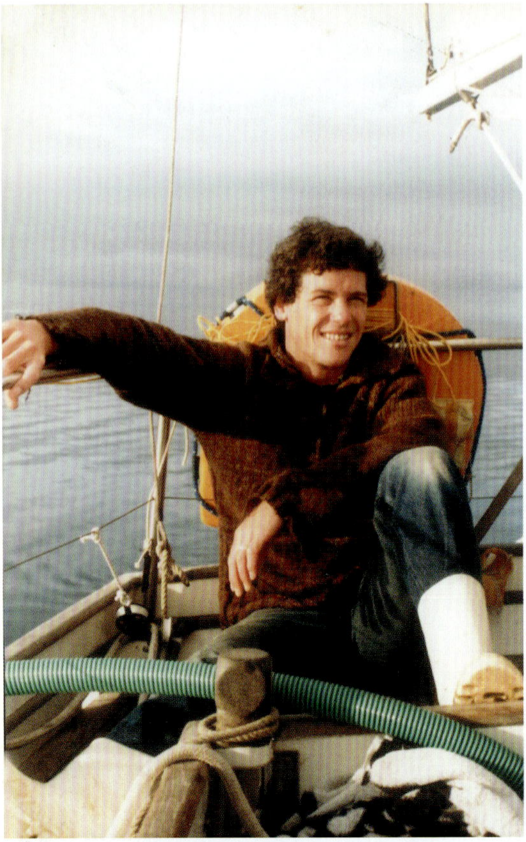

Alistair on Tarua*, 1984.*

With David on Tarua *in a gale, 1985.*

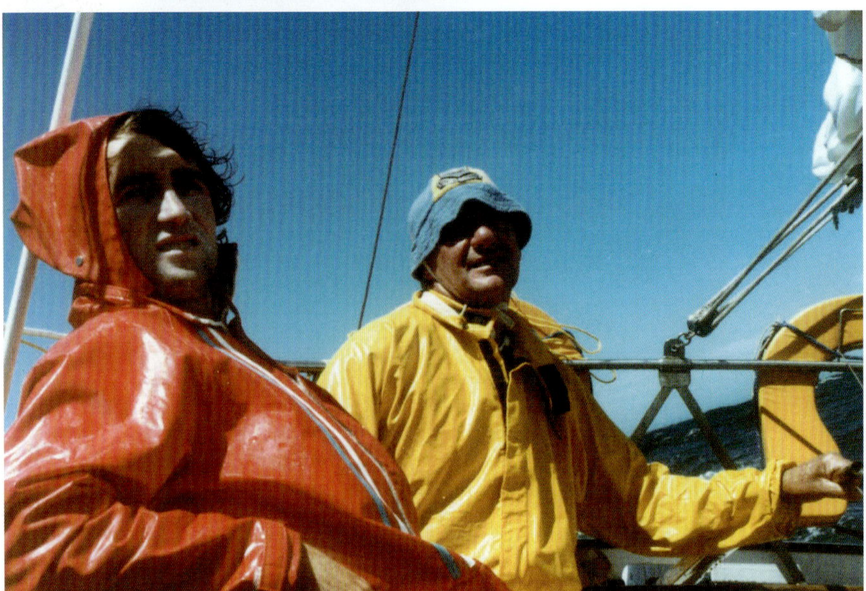

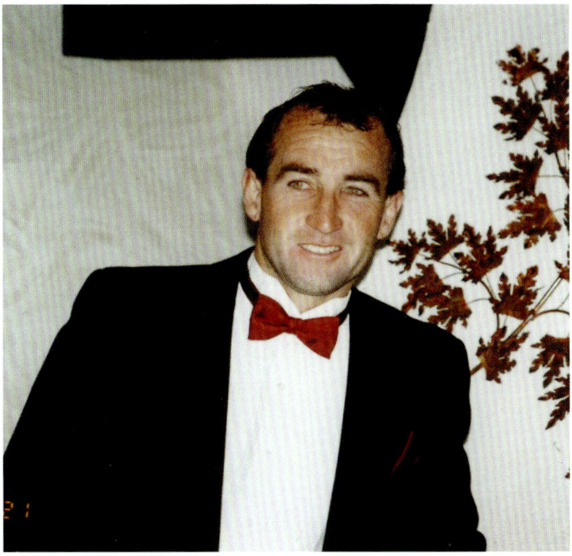

David, 1991.

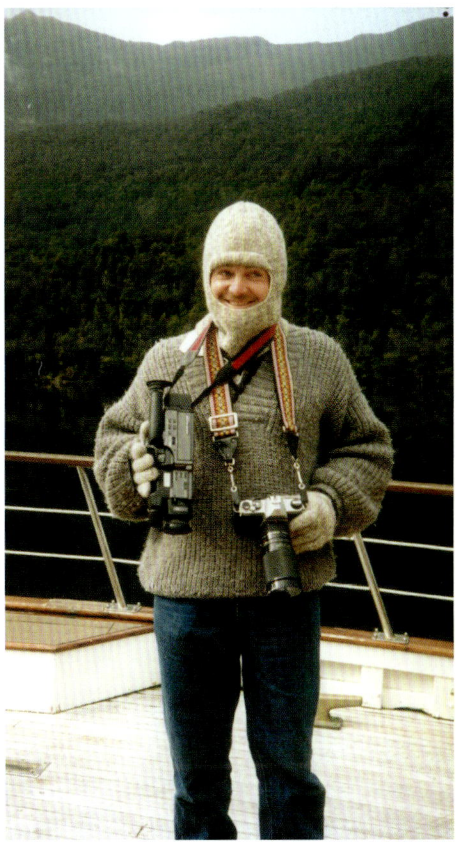

Andrew on Manaia, *Dusky Sound, September 1991.*

Jan, 1993 – captain of the Wellington Representative Hockey Team, winner of the National Hockey Tournament.

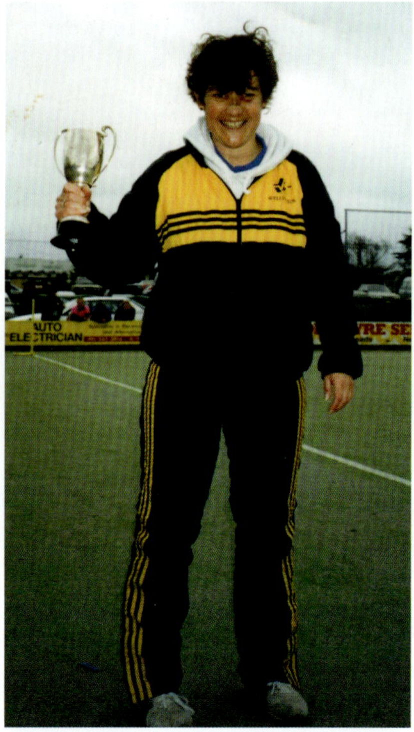

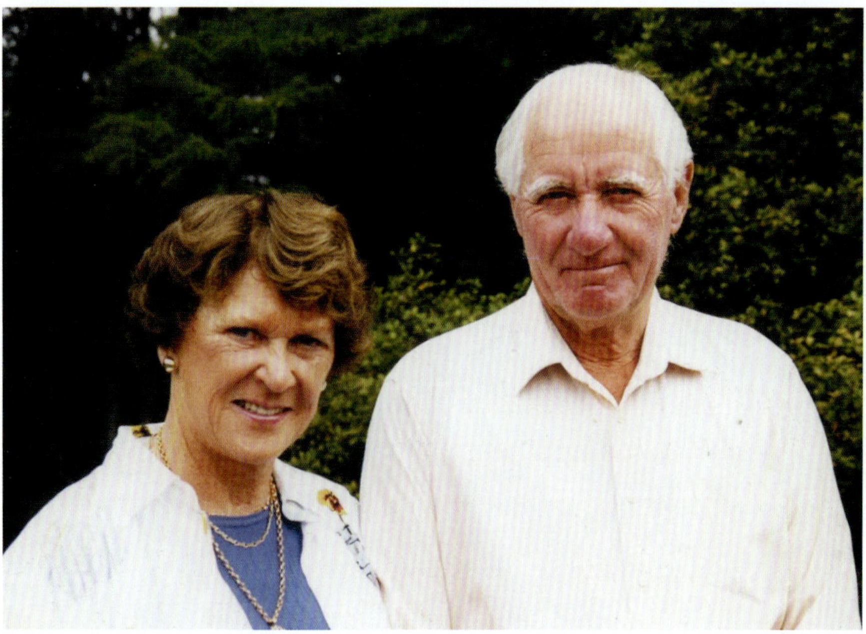

With Joy at End Farm, 1996.

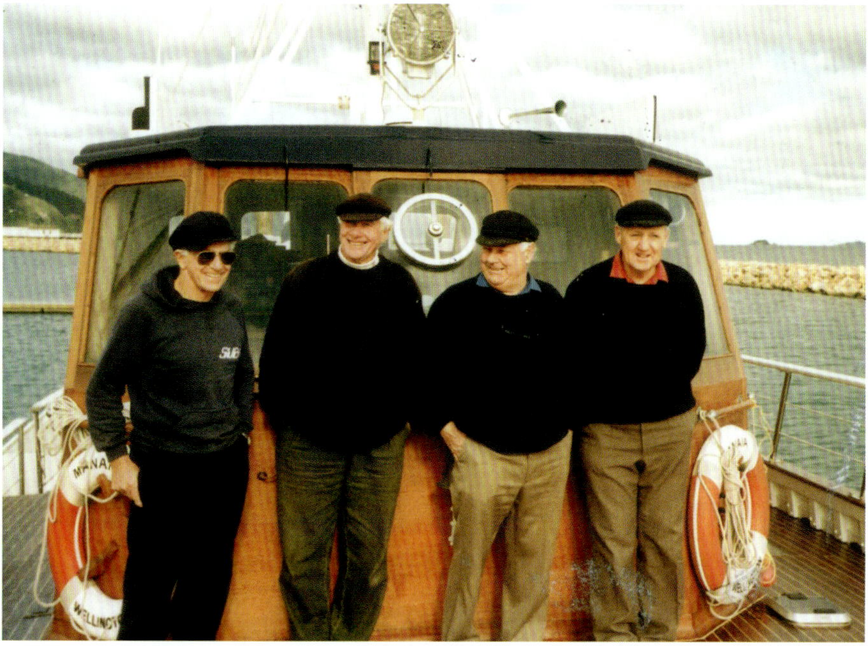

The crew of Manaia *just before sailing for Tonga, 1993.*

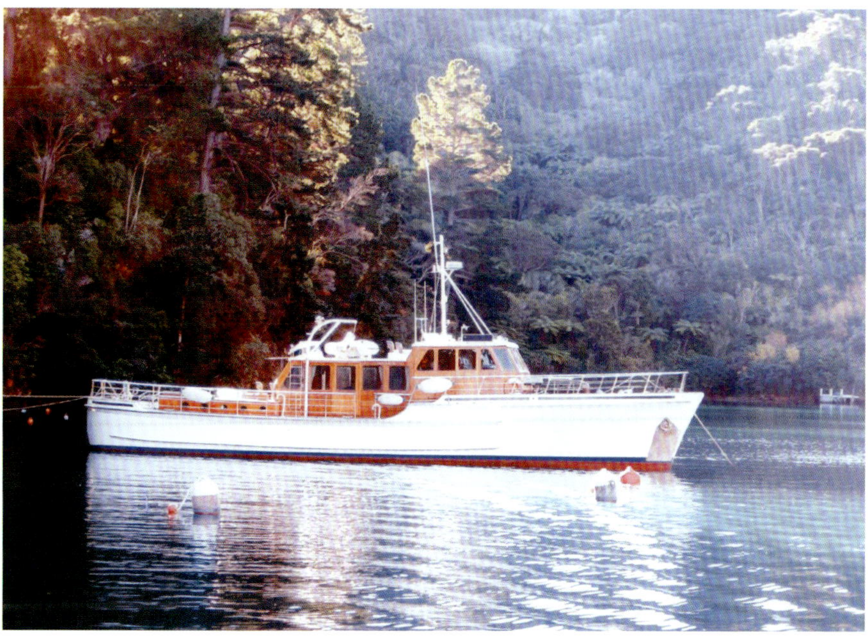

Manaia *in Queen Charlotte Sound, 2005.*

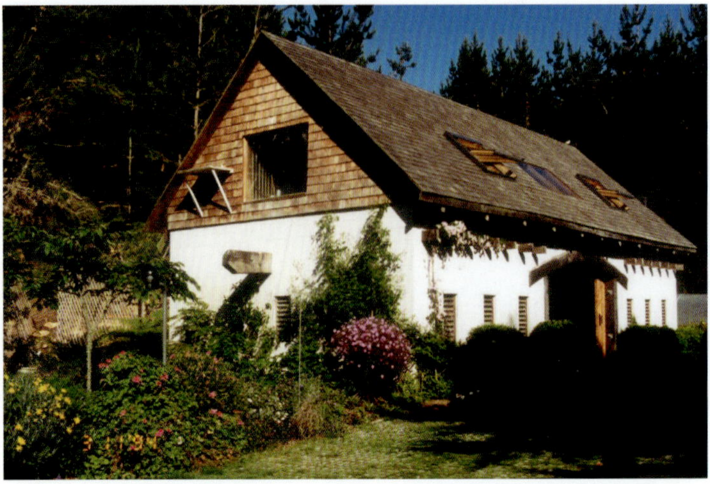

The barn I built at End Farm with Laurie Nicholson, 1988.

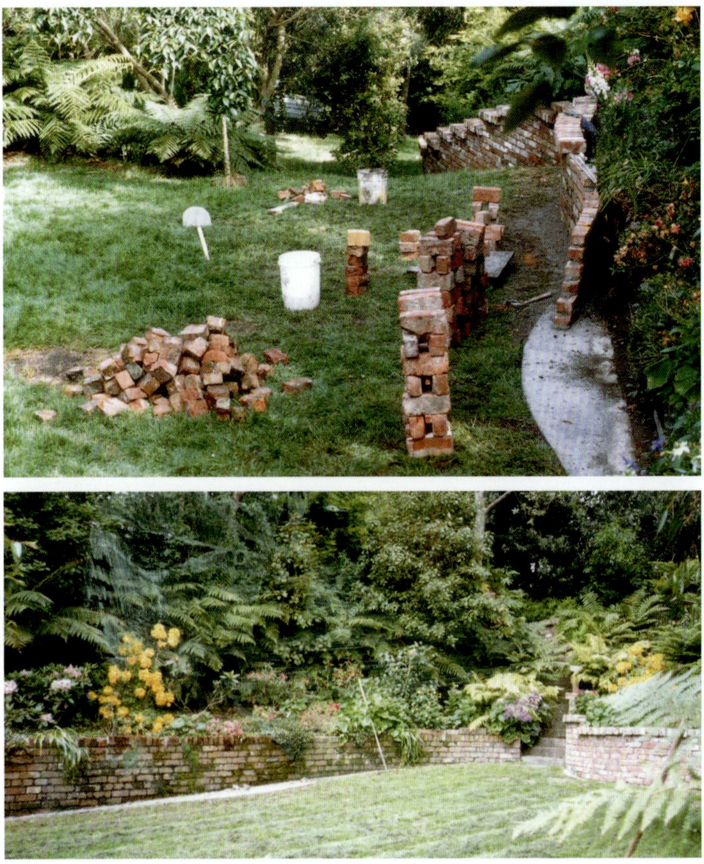

The brick walls under construction (1979–86) and the end result.

too much about it. It is caused simply by postural overstretching of normal ligamentous structures surrounding the disc.

The next stage is reached when eventually the strain on the disc from prolonged sitting or bending becomes excessive and the supporting ligaments tear. Then, instead of disappearing with movement as usual, the pain remains and may increase if displacement of the disc increases at the site of the tearing. Eventually the pain will subside as healing occurs. The final stage is reached when after several recurrences of the damage or tearing, the resultant contracted scar tissue prevents normal movement and perpetuates pain.

The classification of patients in this manner, indicating specific appropriate treatment, had not been possible until now. Patients with disc displacement (derangement syndrome) could be treated and educated with specific exercises that reversed that process; those with scarring from previous disc injury (dysfunction syndrome) could be educated to exercise to stretch and remodel the scar without causing further damage, and those with postural syndrome required nothing more than education to correct their sitting posture. While this became clearer to me by the day, I was preoccupied with my patients and busy practice and I was completely unaware that my conclusions would represent a significant advance in the diagnosis and self-treatment of spinal problems.

Repetitive movements that influenced pain intensity and location were therapeutic if applied appropriately. I soon found out that repeated movements were also diagnostic. Shortly after this a patient came to see me who had been suffering with back pain. On this particular day he was not experiencing any pain at all. If a patient had no pain there was really nothing to work on and it was impossible to identify which movements were detrimental and which were beneficial. But I now had the benefit of so many patterns to draw on and began by asking the patient if he was worse when doing a lot of bending in the garden. The answer was yes and I asked him to bend forward five or six times. He felt uncomfortable after that exercise and I decided that I would see if I could increase the pain and told him to bend, touching his toes, 10 or 12 more times. I became quite excited when he said his pain was gradually increasing. I had induced pain using repeated flexion movements in a patient who prior to that had been symptom free. That seemed a useful technique for diagnosis. It dawned on me that if I could reverse that situation I would have enormously strengthened the case for extension treatment. I was absolutely thrilled, and relieved, when he recovered completely by doing the extension exercises.

I now found I could consistently increase symptoms in some patients by having them repeatedly bend forwards. This immediately indicated the movements that the patient should avoid, as well as identifying the movements that would be beneficial and lead to recovery. The disc model theory was becoming validated by the results achieved by my own experimental work. It was now evident that internal derangement could be clinically induced and reduced simply by repeatedly moving the patient in the wrong direction and then reversing the displacement by repeatedly moving the patient in the corrective direction. In many patients, but not all, it appeared to be a rapidly reversible disorder.

I could predict from a patient's description of how their pain behaved what needed to be done and in which direction they should be exercising, and so often the treatment proved successful. As long as I visualized how the disc might be affected by various movements and positions, solutions in various situations immediately sprang to mind. It all seemed so logical. I developed a range of treatment positions. For example, women who had developed back pain during or after pregnancy seemed frequently to be affected by the posture adopted during pregnancy that increases the hollow in the lower back. They would have difficulty bending forward into flexed positions. I found that rather than recovering with extension (backward) exercise, they rapidly changed with flexion (forward bending) exercises. So it seemed that the disc could bulge forward and inhibit the ability to flex. The disc theory lent support to this.

I continued to find new subtle manoeuvres that induced changes in patients' symptoms. I noted that some patients who did not respond to the push-up exercise did respond positively when the position of their hips was changed. This became a routine part of treatment for patients whose pain was to one side or radiating to the buttock or leg as in the case of sciatica. It was amazing really – if a patient did not respond to routine extension exercises, a simple adjustment achieved by moving the pelvis away from the side of the pain would alter the internal mechanics in such a way that push-ups suddenly became effective. The patient's symptoms would first centralize, then reduce, and finally disappear.

I kept very basic records in those days – the patient's responses to the questions: Where is the pain? How long have you had it? What caused it? Does it ever stop? Are you getting better, worse, or is it unchanging? What happens when you bend forward? What happens when you bend backwards? What happens when you sit, walk and lie down? I diligently recorded the effects of the movements in different directions. I recorded what happened to pain over time when a patient maintained the same posture, where the pain started, and where it moved to.

Checking my records at some point, I noticed that patients with only back pain reported that as they exercised in extension their pain would gradually become less widespread, reduce or disappear, but those who had additional pain in the buttocks or leg reported that the pain in the leg would ease and move towards the mid-line of the spine. This was exactly the sequence described by Mr Smith during his rapid cure. I then knew I should watch for a shift of pain during treatment in all my patients. The shift was occurring in many cases. It was sometimes very rapid in effect, and was always a feature in those who recovered completely. Sometimes it would occur at the first treatment, or gradually over several days. I knew, however, that if the pain was moving towards the middle of the back, no matter how slowly, the patient would get better. I called it "centralization." I don't know why it took me two or three years to recognize the predictability of this.

And, yes, there were failures too. My patients did not always improve and the pain some experienced was aggravated by the exercises. Failure provided a real challenge. I noted that in those with sciatica or pain in the back spreading to the leg there was a consistent pattern in the pain shift – they would describe that it started near the middle of the back and as it worsened the pain would spread and move to one side, then to the buttock and then down the leg. In some patients with sciatica there was no improvement; it was very easy to worsen their problem unless care was taken. It was essential to stop the exercises at the first sign of pain moving further into the buttock or leg. I recorded everything very carefully and realized that this was the exact opposite to the centralization of pain that I was endeavouring to achieve with the exercises. Was it the result of the disc gradually displacing further and eventually compressing the sciatic nerve? Pain moving away from the mid-line therefore could indicate that the condition was worsening. Did this indicate that the disc was displaced excessively and unable to be corrected? Recognition of this turning point was very important because it gave me a warning and a safety alarm. If a patient indicated that his pain was moving outwards or downwards I knew that the exercise I was giving was inappropriate. I referred to this as 'peripheralising pain'. I was now confident in advising patients to avoid any movement that peripheralized their symptoms and choose instead those positions and movements that centralized the symptoms. I became more certain than ever that these phenomena could only be explained by the movement of the disc. So my experimentation went on and many positions, exercises and combinations were found that helped individual patients.

Sciatic scoliosis is a condition that causes the patient to bend to one side, with pain radiating into the leg. My first encounter with a patient with a severe lateral shift was intriguing enough but did not lead to a rapidly successful outcome. The patient was tall and lean and appeared to be bent sideways to the left. He was experiencing quite severe pain in his back and right thigh. I was at a loss to know what to do. I tried to have him do the extension push-ups on the treatment table but he complained that this increased the pain in his buttock. While he was still in the lying position I tried to manoeuvre his upper body so that it was straight. This was successful, but once he stood erect he again slumped to one side. I lay him down again and in this position he could be straightened, but when he stood the deformity reappeared. He could not continue to lie on the table because of pain so I had him stand again. I wondered what would happen if I just pushed him so that he would straighten up. I put my arms around him and squeezed his upper trunk. His body moved slowly in response to this pressure and then suddenly he was bent to his right. He told me he now felt the pain on the other side of his back and left leg. His symptoms and deformation had completely changed sides. He was now in considerably more pain than when he arrived so, although concerned, I could only send him home.

This encounter caused me to consider the possibility that this patient's deformity was also caused by displacement of the disc but in this case a very mobile displacement that could move from side to side. I later realized that the more likely explanation was that the displacement was a fixed displacement in the mid-line and the vertebrae above tilted over that from one side to the other. A few months later I had another patient with almost identical symptoms. I knew that trying to correct the problem in the lying position was ineffectual. I therefore moved the patient to the straight position while he was standing, being careful not to overcorrect. I then bent him backwards into extension. Almost immediately he said his pain had lessened. I repeated this process a few times and he became progressively more mobile and pain free.

I theorized that perhaps the condition could alter in standing but not in the lying position only because of the compression forces that existed with the patient standing. Thus any displacement of the disc would be squeezed more effectively towards the normal. After successfully treating many patients with similar symptoms, I confidently wrote up my discoveries and methods for publication. In spite of my inadequacies in the field of scientific reporting, the paper, "Manual Correction of Sciatic Scoliosis" was accepted for publication by the *New Zealand Medical Journal* in 1972.

Over some ten years, the similarities of patient groups and their responses began to clarify. I also began to recognize that the methods applicable to the lower back were effective in patients with neck problems, and it seemed clear to me that most people with back and neck pain could be successfully treated with selected exercises, positions and restrictions on activity for short periods to allow repair. Many with back problems were being sent off for surgery, and I increasingly believed that very few actually needed such serious intervention. Surgery is itself an injury and should be a last-resort treatment. It was appropriate for those with severe compression of the nerve root that could not be quickly relieved by exercise or re-positioning, but the tendency for surgery to be performed on patients, especially sportspeople who had never been adequately managed non-surgically, increasingly concerned me. I was convinced that until the natural healing process has been given a chance to repair the injury, surgical intervention should not be considered.

By 1965 I was generally pleased with my progress in sorting out some of the common problems I was seeing in Kelvin Chambers. The disc model theory was working very well for me.

CHAPTER 6

HOME LIFE AND THE TURF WAR

Our daughter Jan was 18 months old when our first son, David, arrived in January 1959. At six weeks of age he developed the same pyloric stenosis symptoms I had had early in my life. Following much less radical surgery than mine, David recovered within a few days. Now that there were four of us we again sought to move. The exposed site on top of a hill where we had built our house caught the full force of the prevailing winds, which near Wellington were almost constant, and seeking relief from this, we moved to the Hutt City, at the northern end of Wellington Harbour, which was more sheltered, being on a plain between hills. The house had nice grounds and a garden. Here Joy and I began a shared life-long passion for gardening.

In April 1960 Alistair was born, so we moved again, to a five-bedroom house in the centre of Lower Hutt. In 1963 we welcomed a third son, Andrew, who, at six weeks of age developed the same symptoms of projectile vomiting as had occurred in both his brother David and myself. To have two children develop pyloric stenosis was statistically most unlikely. Andrew, too, rapidly recovered after surgery. Family life provided great pleasures and of course kept us constantly busy. As we had always thought that having a dog around the home was important for children, we now acquired a puppy, a Corgi we named Teddy. Shortly afterwards there would be Teddy Two.

Before I had fully developed my own treatment methods I had also been interested in spinal manipulation. In 1954, shortly after I began in practice, Brian Mulligan, a fellow practitioner in Wellington, and I had decided to teach ourselves some of the techniques. Initially we used Cyriax's books, as he was known to be one of the few doctors championing the cause of physiotherapy. I later learned more from Dr Alan Stoddard. Stoddard was an osteopath at Brook Hospital in London and was the author of *A Manual of Osteopathic Techniques*. We were also given instruction in osteopathic procedures from Stanley Paris, a New Zealand-trained physiotherapist who had spent some time with Stoddard. Paris later published his own book *The Spinal Lesion*. I later visited Dr Stoddard in the UK.

We also had the benefit of instruction in spinal manipulation by Cyriax's chief physiotherapist, Miss Jennifer Hickling, who was in New Zealand for several months in the mid-1950s. We were very good at getting the 'clicks' after a year or so. Gradually, our small local interest group grew. Mulligan and I were joined over the next few years by several colleagues from nearby cities.

During my first years in practice we became aware of the looming threat to our profession from chiropractors, who were gaining recognition and competing for our patients. Some of their patients in New Zealand also began to press for legislation recognising the chiropractors in the national healthcare scheme. As that pressure grew, so also did our opposition to the chiropractors as we attempted to strengthen and protect our profession.

In the late 60s Brian Mulligan and I, along with a few others interested in the method, founded the New Zealand Manipulative Therapists Association (NZMTA) to counter the legislative push. I was elected the first president and was also appointed senior lecturer in manipulation. Brian Mulligan was appointed an instructor. Our first Secretary was Craig Cameron, who had commenced practice in Lower Hutt. (Craig was one of the five males in our first year in the physiotherapy school in Dunedin.) Our objective was to train physiotherapists in spinal manipulation. Our strategy was to demonstrate to the politicians that there was already a manipulative therapy service available for doctors wishing to prescribe that treatment and therefore no need to recognize the chiropractors as they were not the sole providers of manipulation. We formed an alliance with the New Zealand Medical Association. Agreement was reached that the Medical Association would support this rationale.

In 1968 a meeting with Prime Minister Keith Holyoake was organized by Sir Charles Burns, a senior cardiologist in Wellington and a leader in the medical establishment at the time. I attended that meeting with several colleagues from the Private Practitioners' Association. Sir Charles put the case to the Prime Minister in no uncertain terms, calling chiropractic a cult with no scientific evidence to support it and told Holyoake that he was out of step and should in no way encourage quackery! The response was typical of Holyoake: 'I would have you know, Sir Charles, that politics is the highest calling in the land and I am not here to listen to this biased petition.' End of meeting.

As senior lecturer in the NZMTA I was able to introduce my disc theory and procedures. I was now subgrouping patients and using repetitive end-range movement that caused centralization, and I was seeing a reduction or abolition of symptoms in over 70 per cent of them. I was trying to promote these methods among colleagues and others but was discouraged by the lack of interest and disillusioned that so many of my fellow physios and relied almost entirely on spinal manipulation.

I became increasingly dismayed that the direction the NZMTA was taking was leading to the creation of a third profession whose main aim in treatment was the delivery of spinal manipulation. Chiropractors and osteopaths were already well established in this field. The problem as far as I was concerned was that chiropractors relied almost totally on X-rays to make their diagnosis. X-rays were notoriously unreliable and could not positively identify the source of pain in the majority of patients. What was worse, however, were the well publicized claims that chiropractic adjustments could cure visceral and systemic diseases. Osteopaths were also providing manipulation as their main treatment and they relied mostly on what they thought they could feel with their ultra-sensitive fingers. They were also dismissive of the intervertebrate disc as the source of back pain and therefore treated such pain mainly with spinal manipulation.

When the NZMTA decided to follow the osteopathic philosophy and diagnose by 'feel', I was extremely disappointed, as by this time, some nine or ten years after Mr Smith, I was achieving remarkable success in reducing and abolishing low back pain and had deep convictions of the soundness of the disc model theory. What had begun as a 'turf war' became for me a fundamental opposition to the dominance of methods that so often failed to achieve the best outcome for patients.

To this day the NZMTA continues to teach palpatory methods of diagnosis and treatment that long ago lost credibility. Many studies have shown that identifying by feel spinal joints that move excessively or are limited in motion is just not feasible or reliable. Manipulative therapists are always on the lookout for the 'magic bullet'. Whenever some new procedure for manipulating the spine is announced, they flock to see how this is done. It is a burgeoning industry, but the obsession with techniques of manipulation relegates the therapist to the role of a mere technician.

A few years later, about 1970, the Government determined that a Royal Commission of Inquiry would decide the chiropractic status issue. I saw Scott Haldeman, a prominent US leader in the chiropractic political arena, for the first time at the Inquiry. He was an advocate for chiropractic and a very persuasive figure. We did not speak then, but we are now good friends. In 1978 the Commission eventually found in favour of the registration of chiropractors. The rest is history. Chiropractic is recognized as an official health service and treatment costs for chiropractic treatments are now paid for by the New Zealand Accident Compensation Corporation. The turf war was to continue for many years.

Our property in Lower Hutt actually had a 'commercial' zoning, but it was perfect for our needs and would only become more valuable in time. It did not take long, however. One day, about three years after our purchase, there was a knock on the door and we were made an offer made for the property we could not refuse. So the old five-bedroomed house became a funeral parlour and we moved our family once again, this time to a wooded suburb in Silverstream, not far from the old hospital where my career had begun.

Joy had taken up badminton and was playing regularly in competitions. I had been playing an occasional round of golf with one of the locals and became very enthusiastic about it. It provided both relaxation and exercise, which I had been missing. The pity was that I could never predict what would happen to the ball after I had struck it – if I struck it! I got my handicap down to 18 for a few months but that seemed to be as good as it was going to get. I joined the Wellington Golf Club where several of my old friends were members. David Wright, Warren Austad, Clive Stephenson, Peter Hunter, Bill Miles and myself would join up twice a year and visit golf courses in many parts of the North Island. Our "safaris" were enthusiastically anticipated.

All three of our boys were now at the Silverstream primary school and Jan was attending a girls' college in Lower Hutt.

During these busy years I also developed an interest in art. In 1961, while out of curiosity watching Dunbar Sloane's art auction in Wellington during a lunch break, I was taken with a large oil painting of a lake in the South Island and found myself raising my hand at 90 pounds and becoming the proud owner of a painting by W.G. Baker, circa 1850.

We enthusiastically collected further early New Zealand paintings, most of which had been painted by surveyors in their exploration of the new colony of New Zealand and captured the spectacular scenery they encountered. Other works featured the sailing ships that brought the first immigrants from England at that time. These were of little or no interest to the connoisseurs of the art world and were sold very reasonably. Ten years later interest in early New Zealand art exploded and prices skyrocketed.

On one of my auction-room forays, about 1970, I was attracted by a painting of a knight in armour lying on his coffin with arms crossed over his sword. It was painted in oils on a slab of wood and was apparently very old. An inscription, written on the back in Old English, read "The death of Tossarelli". It was painted by Cypriani. I bought the painting for $25. On researching the name of the artist, I found that he was quite famous and became convinced – in spite of Joy's reservations – that I had found a lost masterpiece.

I wrote to Sotheby's, the famous art auction house in London, described the painting and enquired as to the interest they might have in selling it at auction. I became very excited when the reply came back to advise that some paintings by the same artist had fetched as much as five hundred thousand pounds. They were of course much larger and painted on canvas. Sotheby's advised that they would not be able to put a price on Cypriani's "Tosarelli". Did this mean it was priceless? Joy did not think so. Still undaunted I had the painting insured at a cost of $150 and posted it special delivery to London, a further $10.

The painting would be auctioned as lot 155 in September 1971. This coincided brilliantly with a trip we had planned to Monte Carlo. It would be wonderful to be at the auction. Joy and I entered Sotheby's auction rooms full of excitement just five minutes before Lot 155 was put up for sale. There were only three bids. Tosarelli was sold for 25 pounds sterling. We lost a lot of money on that damned piece of wood!

During the mid-60s my good friend Keith Ritson had become quite ill and spent the last few years of his life carrying an oxygen bottle to help him breathe. He asked me if I would take on the responsibility of fee negotiations for the Society. I did so for six years, until further significant changes allowed private clinics to set their own fees without government subsidy.

In 1970, when Keith died, his wife, Noeline, approached me for advice on what to do with her late husband's practice. She had invited another physiotherapist to take over temporarily and look after the many patients. He saw the great opportunity and offered to buy the practice for $3,000. Noeline asked my opinion of its worth and I told her it was worth $4,000–$5,000 and persuaded her to stick to a price in this area. She did so, but the miffed therapist threatened to leave the patients unattended. I offered Noeline $5,000 for the practice and suggested she tell the bloke to go to hell! I found someone else to run Keith's clinic and it continued to do very well. I hired Noeline and she worked in my clinic as my practice nurse and receptionist for the next 15 years.

Throughout the 1960s I had become very accustomed to the rapid and positive changes I so frequently saw in my patients and was very confident of the disc theory. I considered that the best way to convince others of the efficacy of the treatment was to demonstrate with live patients, but very few clinicians were prepared to give up the time to come to my clinic to observe. I also hoped that the local physicians would be enthusiastic enough to study the effects further but I could not find anyone in New Zealand in orthopaedics who had the interest or expertise to undertake an investigation. They were all preoccupied with their own surgery. In any case my claim that I could very often transfer a patient's leg pain to his back was greeted with scepticism.

The world seemed not ready to listen, so in 1968 I was surprized to be invited by the New Zealand Orthopaedic Association to speak at their annual meeting. They even offered to pay my travel and accommodation at The Chateau, a luxury resort just south of Lake Taupo. I immediately accepted this invitation, excited by this unexpected opportunity to tell my story.

I prepared a 30-minute lecture as requested. I arrived with my presentation and a box of slides with an hour to spare, but on reading the programme I was horrified to see that I had been actually allocated only ten minutes. In panic I tried to condense my presentation but had only managed to get halfway through it when a red light signalled the end of my presentation. I was able to tell the gathering only that many patients with leg pain could be successfully managed without surgery, and that extension exercise and certain lateral modifications could abolish symptoms in minutes in some cases. There were no questions at all, but that evening at the conference dinner a young surgeon rather aggressively challenged me, saying that what I had told them was just too good to be true and that I should have some independent confirmation to offer an audience. They never did pay my expenses! This opportunity had certainly ended in failure and I was devastated.

And matters only got worse. Shortly afterwards a patient was referred to me by one of Wellington's most respected and senior orthopaedic surgeons, Kennedy Elliot. He had attended the Chateau conference. He ordered that the patient have heat, massage and exercises for back pain, the routine prescription from this surgeon. Upon examination I recognized that she was an ideal candidate for my new approach of re-positioning and exercise and, indeed, she responded quickly and completely. However, when she returned to the doctor for a follow-up appointment and reported how I had treated her, I received a very terse phone call from him telling me that I had brought myself into disrepute and as far as he was concerned I would stay that way. He would certainly never send me another patient! He then reported me to the New Zealand Physiotherapy Society and asked that I be disciplined. The president of the society at the time was Barbara Tomlinson. After hearing my view she determined, to my relief, that the doctor's reaction was farcical and took no action. However, that surgeon never referred another patient to me and he talked freely to his colleagues of his discontent with me. Referrals from those orthopaedic surgeons declined for a period.

I now wondered if my treatment methods would ever be taken seriously. At this time in New Zealand the orthopaedic surgeons prescribed every detail of the treatment to be done by physios, and now that I was achieving such successful outcomes for patients with my treatment, this felt very restrictive. I felt strongly that patients deserved the opportunity to avoid surgery.

The general practitioners in Wellington were more open-minded towards my management of their patients. They did not really mind what methods I used as long as the patients improved. A few local GPs accompanied their problem patients to my clinic and were sufficiently impressed that thereafter they provided me with a never-ending supply of 'bad backs'. It was the support of the GPs in Wellington – David Virtue, Roger Ridley-Smith, Peter Tuckey, Peter Anyon, Ashton Fitchett, Alex King, Geoff Kiddle, Moir Kronfeld – that allowed me to build a substantial practice specializing in spinal disorders.

At the end of the 1960s a few of my fellow therapists from around the country came to observe my methods as well. Some recognized that my system of diagnosis and treatment was better than anything else they had been taught, including spinal manipulation procedures that had absorbed everyone's interest in recent years. Before long there were several colleagues, including Mark Laslett, Ace Neame and Paula van Wijmen, applying the same diagnostic and treatment methods. But even with staunch support from these friends in the profession there was no great clamour from NZMTA or the Physiotherapy Society to learn more.

There was hostility from some in the manipulator fraternity, who felt betrayed that one of their founders had apparently abandoned hands-on spinal manipulation treatments in favour of hands-off methods or even self-treatment, and who also claimed that these methods were more effective than manipulation in most cases. The idea that some patients would become independent of therapy and therapists was threatening. Even today the New Zealand Manipulative Therapists Association does not include my system of Mechanical Diagnosis and Therapy (MDT) in their education programme. Initially this rejection concerned me greatly, but I could only continue what I firmly believed was in the best interests of the patient. My work provided me enormous satisfaction even though spreading the benefits of my discovery was proving to be an impossible task.

CHAPTER 7

BEGINNING THE LONGEST JOURNEY

In 1968, in spite of the failure to have my treatment methods taken seriously or adopted in New Zealand, I decided to travel and visit all of the world-recognized experts for non-surgical spine treatment. I wanted to observe their methods of treatment because I thought that someone else, somewhere, must have discovered centralization and be using similar methods. I considered that if I added new information and procedures to my already successful techniques, I would excel in the treatment of spinal problems.

With Joy's blessing I re-mortgaged our home to pay for this 14-week trip and for the first time left Joy and our four young children to manage alone. I first flew to Vancouver, Canada to talk to Bourdillon and then to Harry Farfan in Montreal. Then I went on to see James Mennell and Stan Paris in the USA, Cyriax and Stoddard in London, Kaltenborn in Oslo, Maigne in Paris and, on the way back, Maitland in Adelaide. Talking to these people, it quickly became evident to me that none of these leading practitioners knew anything about the effects of repeating movements to end range or about centralization, and, furthermore, they didn't seem to want to know. In the United Kingdom my first visit was to James Cyriax, who had stimulated my early thinking on the relationship between discs and back pain. I was able to observe patients who came to Cyriax's clinics. Some attended for six weeks and even longer and I believed I could have helped many of them in one or two days.

After three weeks of observing Cyriax's therapists manipulating people in what I had long ago found to be the wrong direction, I took the bull by the horns and offered to show the great man a film I had made of a patient with sciatic scoliosis, the condition I wrote about in 1972 in the *New Zealand Medical Journal*. The treatment was previously unknown; the film – shot live with a real patient – was a world first. Cyriax was impressed, and indeed he actually included the procedure in the next edition of his book on low back pain, but unfortunately the manoeuvre was incorrectly described in that text and I would be surprised if any patient improved as a result of it. Cyriax was pleased to comment on the value of my treatment method for acute scoliosis, probably because it was associated and derived from his own work on the disc.

My next destination was Freddy Kaltenborn's physiotherapy clinic in Oslo, Norway. Kaltenborn was a very big man with very big hands. He had developed mobilization and manipulation skills to a high level of perfection following osteopathic principles. Most of these were unfamiliar to me as they were not known well or utilized by New Zealand physiotherapists. Osteopaths at that time believed they could direct pressure to one single spinal joint in the middle of several others. They also believed that they could find the precise spot that needed this force by palpating the spinal joints with their fingers. I had serious reservations about the ability to localize manipulation to this degree of accuracy. In fact I did not then, and do not now, believe this to be possible. Many good quality studies have shown diagnosis by 'feel', or more correctly 'palpation', to be unreliable and of little value in determining the origin of back problems.

In Norway I did not see any more effective techniques than mine to treat patients. However, I was very impressed with the organization of their postgraduate education programme in manipulation. Physiotherapists and physicians would come together for several days and would then go back to their clinics to practice and refine the skills they had learned. They would meet again some months later to advance their understandings of various techniques and strategies and to compare notes and experiences. I could see the benefit that learning through a series of exposures to new ideas and practices would offer.

Despite my diminished enthusiasm for manipulation, I thought Kaltenborn's books on the procedures he used were worthy of consideration by the NZMTA and eventually, with Freddy's help, I had them translated into English. But I was frustrated while observing in Freddy Kaltenborn's clinic. Here also they did not exercise patients to affect the disc; they exercised them to strengthen their muscles and, in addition, most patients received manipulation. The exercise procedures I had developed were immediately effective in most patients because they were directed to the joints and discs of the spine. Strengthening muscles had no long-lasting effect on the joints and so had little or no effect on the pain.

Freddy introduced me to one of his associates, Rolf Gustaveson. I visited Rolf and will always remember his saying to me, "The answer to neck problems lies somewhere between here and here", and to show what he meant he moved his head as far as possible forward and then as far as possible backward without tilting the head up or down. I played with that idea with patients attending with neck problems and eventually found that if the movements were repeated to the full possible range they would also affect the location and intensity of pain in the same manner that occurred in the low back. When the head is kept in a forward position or moved forward repeatedly the patient's symptoms would appear to worsen. When the head is held back over the spine the symptoms reduce or cease. This was a very important step forward. Rolf just hadn't worked out how to relate the movement to the pain experience.

Upon my return to New Zealand I pondered what I had seen. I had spent a significant amount of time and money visiting the most reputable non-surgical treatment centres in the world and had come back disappointed. Most of these clinics were using and advocating mobilization or manipulation as the treatment of choice for spine patients, and while a few patients immediately improved as a result, most did not. The method I had discovered and refined was unique; it allowed for identification of subgroups and provided prognostic indication. I was confident and proud of my work but I now despaired of ever being able to demonstrate what I knew outside New Zealand.

My offers to do so while at these clinics were always politely declined. It was a huge predicament; how could I pass on this knowledge and convince people of its effectiveness? How could I persuade people of the real importance of new discoveries in a field that had been dogged by cults, dogma, gurus and quacks since the beginning of time? I was still unable to convince anyone in a position of influence to help me put centralization and mechanical diagnosis and therapy on the map.

I had lost my enthusiasm for manipulative therapy and could not continue to promote and teach manual procedures which were inferior in so many ways to self-applied treatments. Teaching the patient to mobilize himself by applying his own end-range exercise consistently proved so much more effective than manipulation. From the earliest days in practice I had been using manual skills to treat patients, and the 'hands on' approach was universal among therapists involved in treating muscles and joints. The move to a 'hands off' approach was a huge step, but now an increasingly attractive one to me. Some patients were unable to apply enough force on their own, and who still required extra assistance by way of manipulation, but nevertheless I felt we should not be manipulating all patients with spinal pain. This was a new way of working rather than an additional mechanical technique. There was no magic technique that would cure all patients, but understanding the mechanisms of pain generation increasingly seemed fundamental to treatment options. Our profession generally seemed to lack the desire or receptivity to explore this dimension of treatment.

Very early in our marriage we had visited the Marlborough Sounds, a vast area of sunken valleys at the top of the South Island. The beautiful waterways were largely unspoiled and some of the hillsides were still covered in their same native forest that had been there when Captain James Cook discovered the inlets in 1769. The only access through the Sounds was by boat. I had long held a desire to return to this glorious place and slowly the idea of buying a boat for the family grew. Cook Strait separates the two main islands and is subject to severe winds and high seas, so only a sturdy vessel would handle it. Now was the time to sell some of our art collection.

Joy was initially rather dubious about the boat, mainly because I had no sailing experience. Would we be able to manage a yacht with sails and ropes and the often wild weather in the Strait? Throwing caution to the winds, Joy agreed it would be wonderful for the family and gave the idea her full support.

Around 1970, not long after my disappointing European trip, I found what I thought was an ideal vessel: a steel-hulled 40-foot two-masted cruising ketch with two cabins. After a trial sail across Cook Strait to the Sounds with the owner in command – and in perfect weather and flat seas – the deal was done. I had watched the skipper at work and determined that it was really a very simple task to set the sails and go sailing. Why was everyone so cautious about yachting? Joy inspected *Sundance* and gave her approval. Some of the paintings were auctioned and more than enough was realized to enable the purchase of the ketch. The adventure was begun.

For the next six months I attended night classes at the New Zealand Marine Department, studying for and finally earning my yacht-master's ticket. We were planning to spend a few weeks over Christmas and New Year in the Sounds. Learning navigation in the classroom was all rather easy. On the morning of Christmas Eve, amidst great excitement, all six of us set forth from Paremata Harbour, just north of Wellington, to Queen Charlotte Sound – a distance of some 20 miles. I concealed my slight trepidation at the full realization that I was now in sole charge of a vessel, the workings of which I knew little. However, once the sails were up we crossed the Strait in fair weather with no problems. We arrived just on sunset and immediately began to search for a suitable place to anchor. After an hour studying the charts, I managed to identify where we were. I found a sheltered bay and was wondering how to lower the anchor when I spotted a mooring buoy close by. It couldn't have been easier. Satisfied with our luck, I pulled the buoy tight.

Only minor challenges presented themselves on this, our first night on board. After struggling to light the gas stove, we eventually found the tap to turn on the supply and enjoyed our first meal afloat before heading for our beds.

The children, as always, were awake early in the morning and I could hear feet running around the deck. The hatch to our cabin slid open, with David announcing, 'Daddy, we are a long way from shore.' I told him not to be so silly, but hurriedly looked out my side window. It was indeed a long way to the beach. I looked out the opposite side – it was no joke. We didn't appear to be in any danger but I quickly tried to pull the anchor rope in. That was impossible. Embarrassed at this early setback and expecting it might create in the first mate a certain loss of confidence in the skipper, I cut the rope holding us. Immediately the bow raised a couple of feet, having been held down by the weight of whatever was at the end of the rope. I started the engine and moved on as quickly as possible, hoping no one had observed us. Puzzling over what had gone wrong, it finally dawned on me that it was due to my having pulled the mooring tight on arrival. The tide had been out at then, and when the tide came in *Sundance* lifted with it and also lifted the mooring block off the sea floor! We were free to float wherever the wind or tide took us. Fortunately there was little wind that first night. The lesson was learned – never use a mooring without allowing sufficient slack in the chain for a rising tide. My navigation course had not actually covered the use of moorings.

This was just the beginning of a long chapter of incidents that made for wonderful adventures in the Sounds and on the seas for us all.

CHAPTER 8
LONDON, MONTE CARLO AND END FARM

While in London in 1968 I had visited a member of the British Association of Manual Medicine, Dr John Ebbetts. Ebbetts had qualified first as a medical doctor and later as a chiropractor. It was his experience with chiropractic that fostered his desire to establish links between orthodox medicine and alternative therapies.

For a few days I observed Ebbetts treating his patients. Like Dr Cyriax, he also seemed interested in my film of the correction of the acute scoliosis patient and suggested that I return to Europe in 1970 to attend the European Federation of Manual Medicine's annual meeting in Monte Carlo. He wanted me to show the film to the large group at the conference, expected to be about 300 people. I was very excited by his enthusiasm. I did not mention repeated movements or centralization or anything else, thinking the film would be just a start, a foot-in-the-door so to speak, and the other stuff could be revealed later.

The problem was I could not see how I would be able to afford to make another journey half-way around the world so soon after my recent trip, as the payments on our increased mortgage were only just affordable. But that guardian angel appeared out of the blue in another guise. I was still doing some home visits at the time and during one such call I was telling a patient, Moira Todd, about the invitation to show my film at the conference and that I was going to have the film copied and sent over to Monte Carlo. She asked me if I was also going, and when I said I couldn't, she asked why not. Moira paid for Joy and me to travel to Monaco. She was a most remarkable woman. I learned later that after the Vietnam War she had paid for the construction, management and staffing of a children's orphanage in that war-torn country. She had apparently assisted hundreds of people and organizations she believed in. So once again a grateful patient helped me at a turning point in my life and my career.

It was a cloak-and-dagger operation to smuggle me into the conference. The European Federation of Manual Medicine did not actually allow physiotherapists to attend its meetings. John Ebbetts advised me to apply for registration, putting MNZSP after my name, but not to mention that I was a physiotherapist. He was confident that the registration office would think I was a member of the New Zealand Society of Physicians and accept my attendance. They did. Joy and I travelled from London to Monaco with John, his wife, and the British contingent. I was accepted by them and they thought it a huge joke to hoodwink the French organizing committee. However, after the first showing of the film someone drew attention to the fact that some of the equipment visible indicated it was from a physiotherapy clinic. Robert Maigne, the French President of the organization at the time, was not pleased, but nothing was done as the contribution was deemed to be sufficiently important to overlook the breach of security.

My session was scheduled at the same time as that of renowned American doctor James Mennell. As a result, my film attracted just 20 people, while Mennell had an audience of 200 in the main hall next door. That evening the organizers of the conference asked me if I would show the film again the next day – this time in the main hall. Evidently someone who had watched the first showing of the 8mm home movie was a member of the organizing committee and believed my film deserved a bigger audience. The word had spread about the manoeuvre that was immediately effective in correcting a condition commonly encountered by anyone treating back problems. And so the situation of the day before was reversed; almost 200 specialists appeared to watch the film, and some 20 or so went next door to hear Mennell.

This event earned me a certain respect in Europe, but I wondered how many understood the implications of what they had seen. The likely impression was of an isolated case where a physiotherapist had squeezed a man who was all bent over and in pain and within a few minutes he was straight, symptom free and smiling. The film provided no real understanding of the theory or the method. Not one of the physicians at the Monte Carlo meeting seemed to recognize the implications and significance of pain centralization. A diagnostic and treatment method to reliably predict and achieve good outcomes in patients with spinal pain had so far eluded medical science. I knew centralization was the answer, but now realized the message needed more than my simple film could demonstrate.

I was deeply grateful to Cyriax and Ebbetts though, as thanks to them I was quickly, and permanently, associated with this method of correction of acute scoliosis, particularly in the United Kingdom where both doctors practised.

My clinic in Wellington was thriving – over the past decade acceptance of my methods had grown amongst the medical fraternity, with patients also advocating my treatment to others. I now needed to employ someone full-time to help me. My first assistant was Jean Buswell, an immigrant physiotherapist with a very broad Scottish accent. She worked in the clinic for five or so years from 1969. In 1974 Colin Davies replaced Jean, and although only in the clinic for a year, he was to remain a life-long lieutenant.

I continued to teach those who were interested in my methods, which meant that only a small proportion of the therapists in New Zealand knew parts of my approach and were using the principles as well as they could. Others did not seem to like the method and were critical of me because I had once championed spinal manipulation but was now committed to teaching patients to treat themselves. At one of the annual meetings of the NZMTA I had proposed that they embark on a study to compare the results of spinal manipulation treatments with my self-treatment system. The suggestion was immediately rejected by almost the entire membership. One member suggested that I was merely trying to publicize my own approach

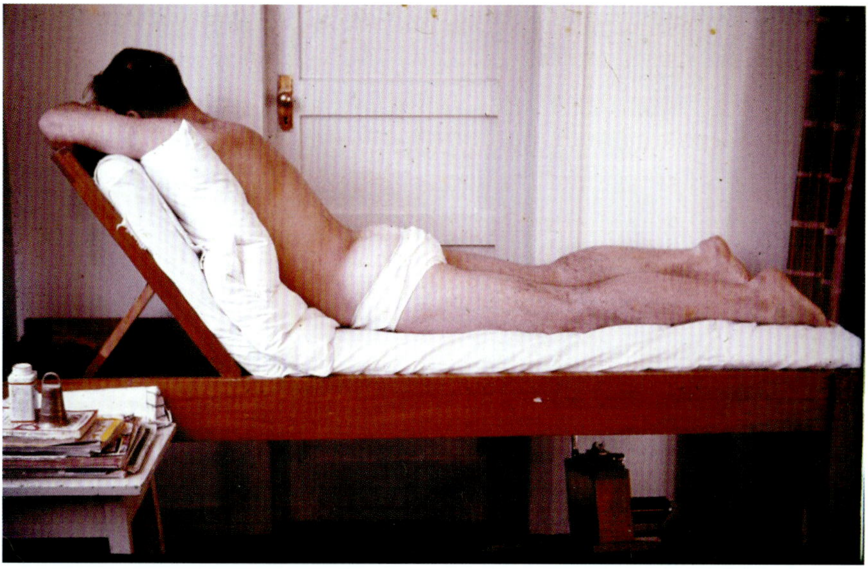

"Mr Smith" lying in extension.

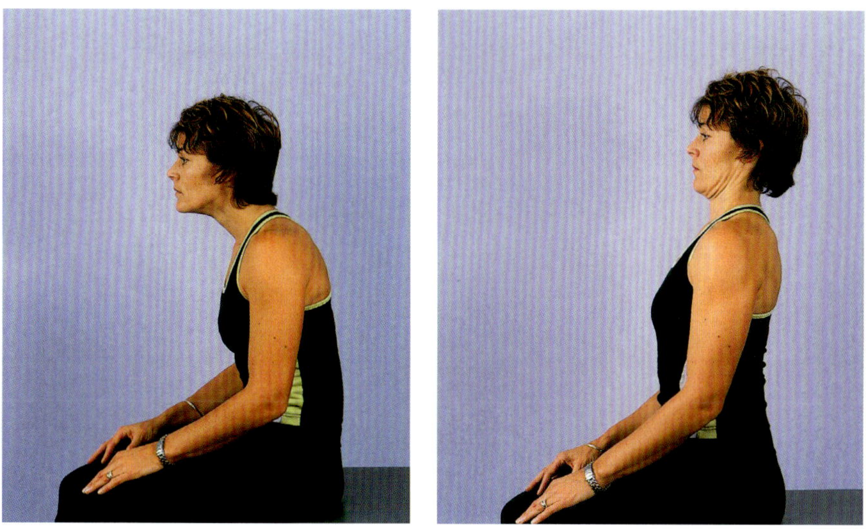

"The answer to pain in the neck lies somewhere between here [left] and here [right]", said Rolf Gustaveson in Norway in 1967.

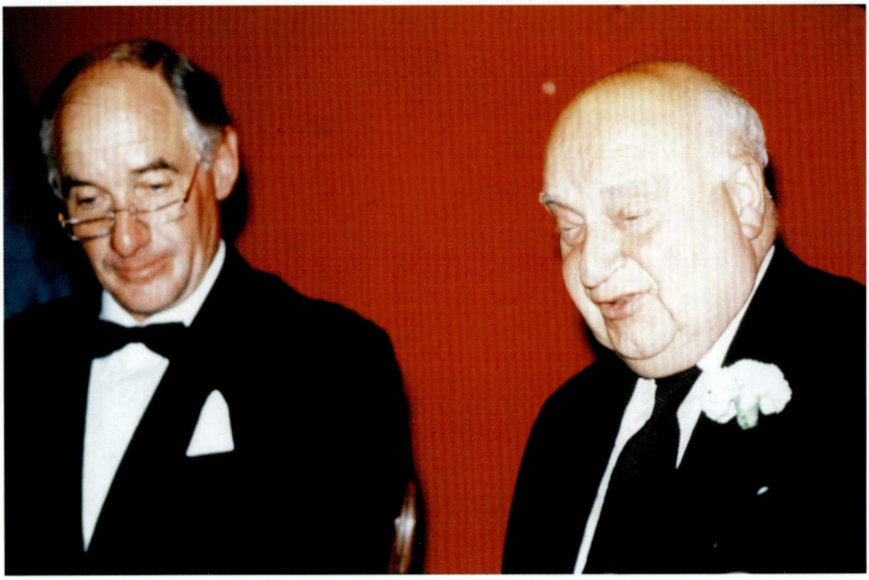

With James Cyriax at a banquet in his honour, Christchurch, 1980.

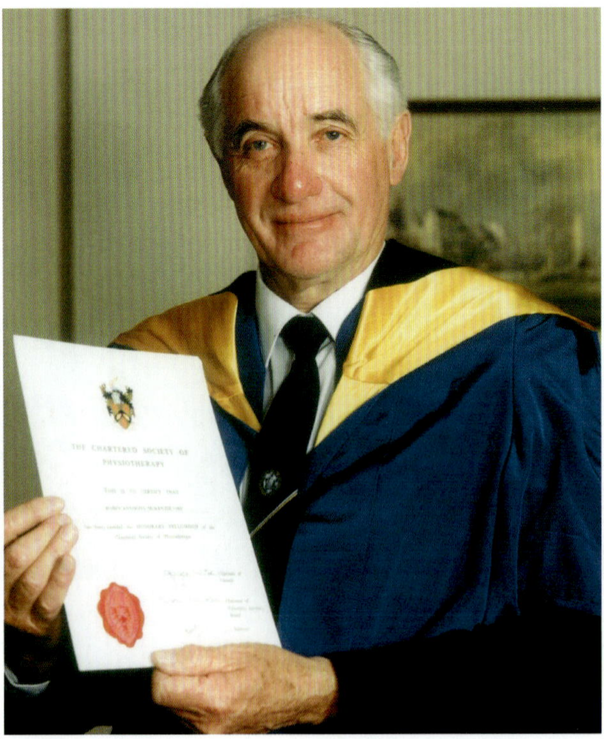

After receiving the Honorary Fellowship of the Chartered Society of Physiotherapy UK in 1990.

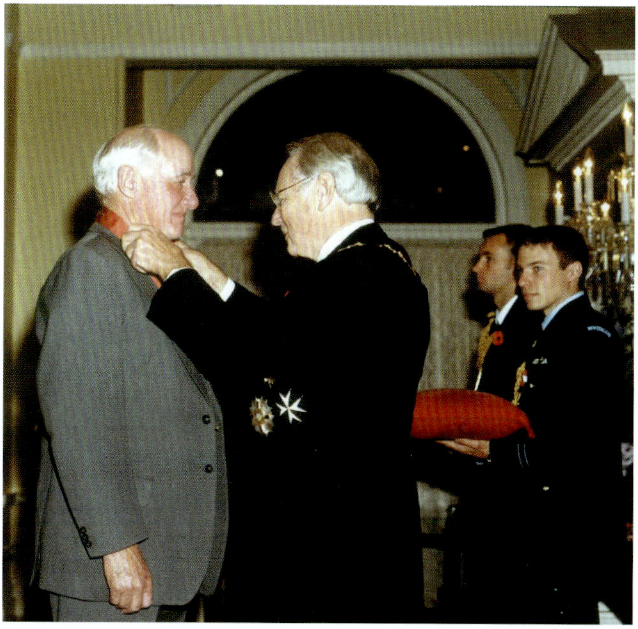

1990 Queen's Birthday Honours – receiving the award of Officer of the Most Excellent Order of the British Empire (OBE) from the Governor General, Sir Michael Hardie Boys.

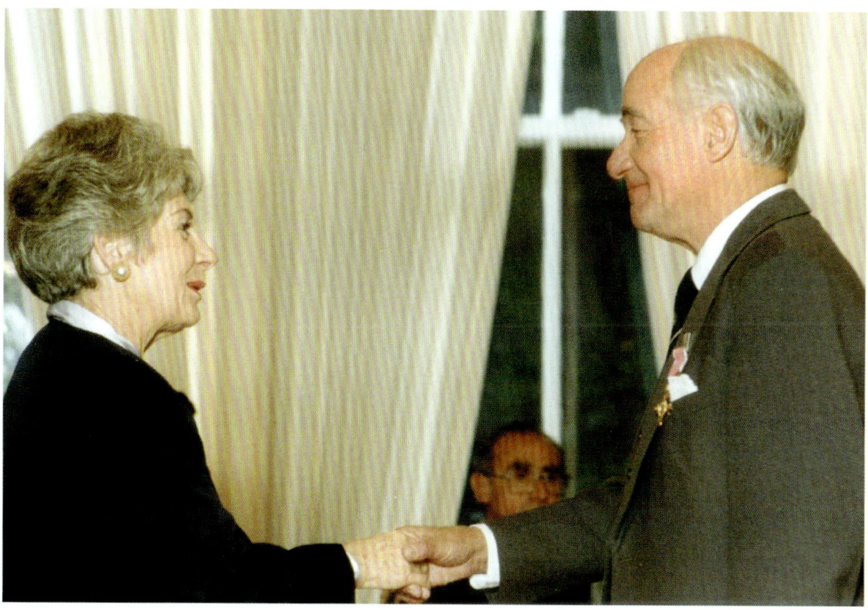

In the New Year's Honours 2000, receiving the Companion of the New Zealand Order of Merit (CNZM) from the Governor General, Dame Kath Tizard.

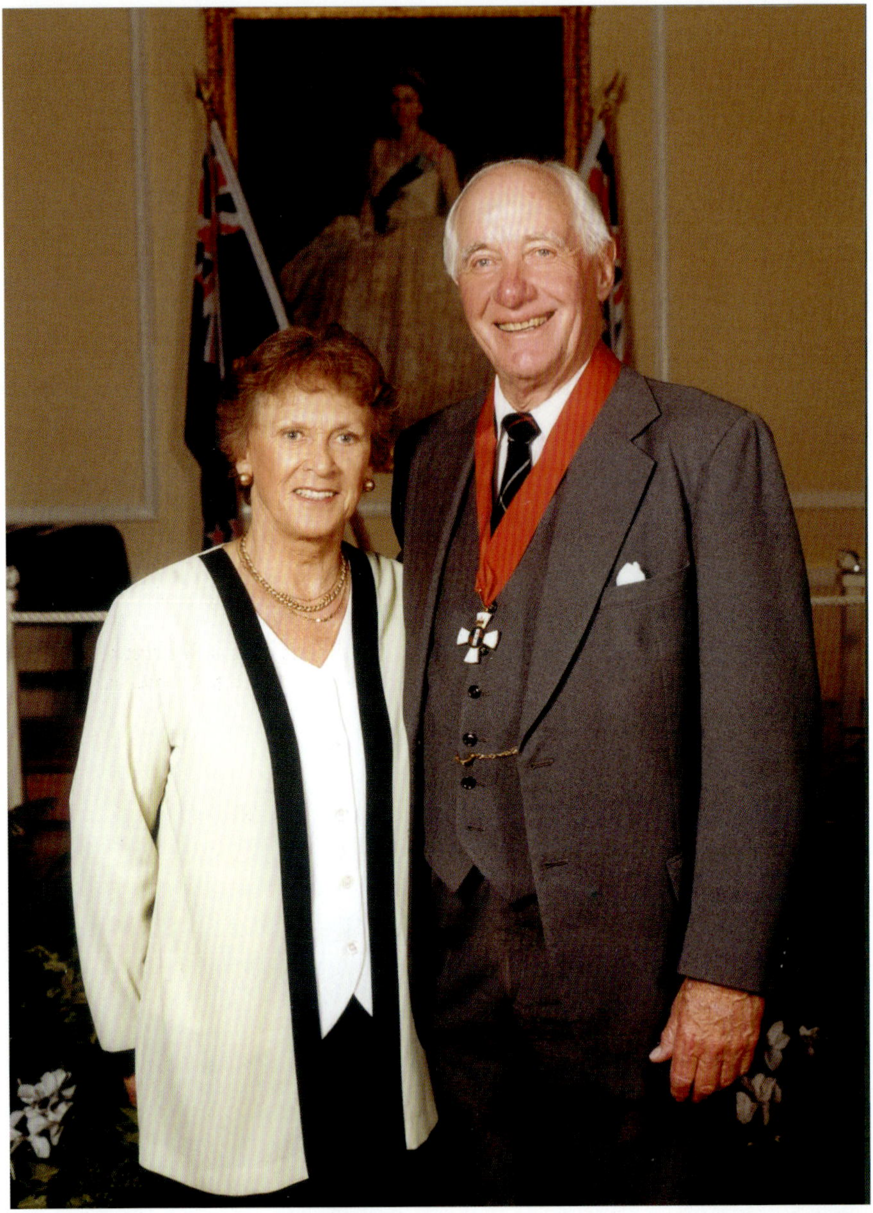

With Joy after receiving the OBE.

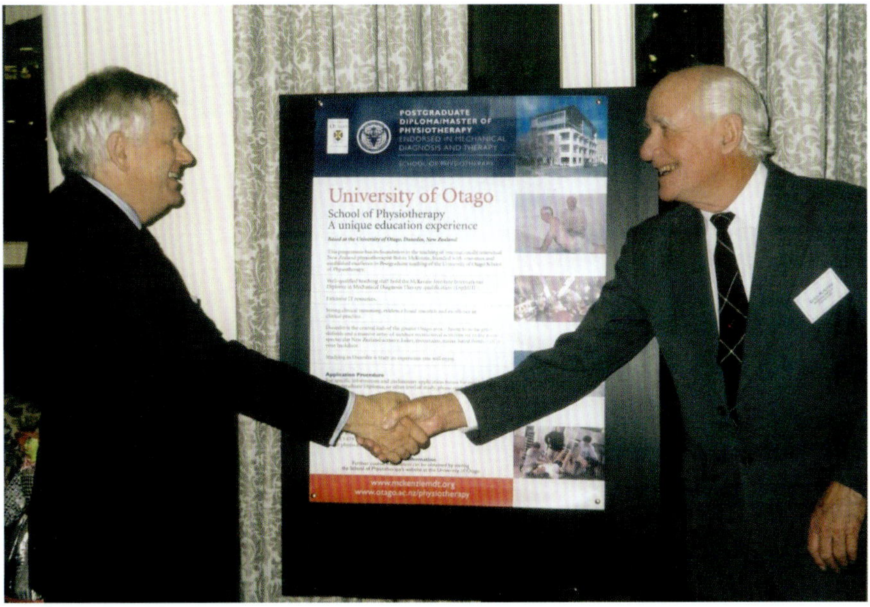

With Vice Chancellor Fogelberg after signing the joint venture agreement between the University of Otago and McKenzie Institute International, 2004.

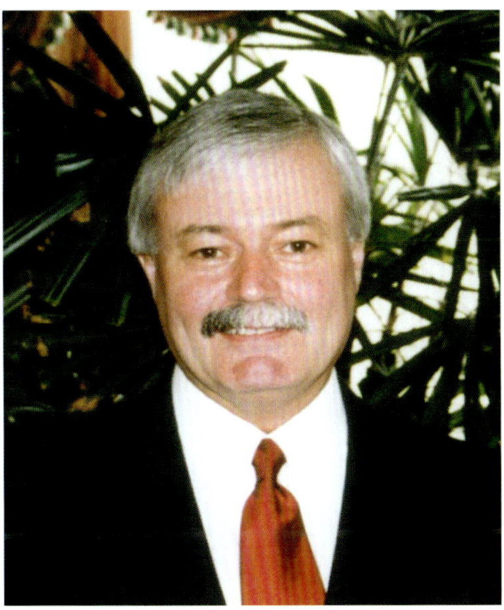

Lawrence Dott. The Institute Chief Executive Officer under whose skilled guidance MDT *continues to expand worldwide.*

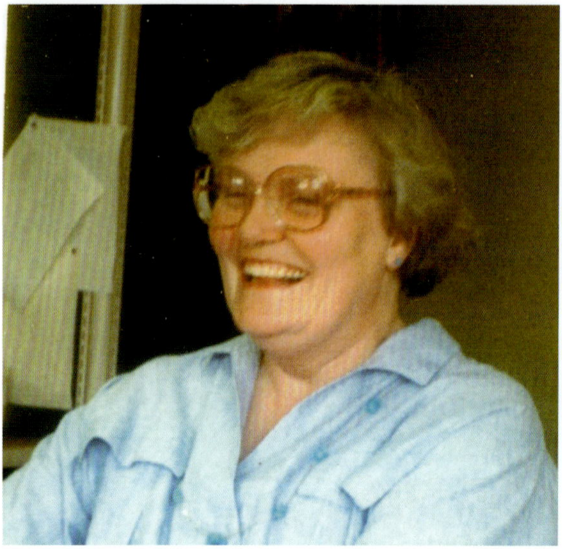

Joanne Moffat, my secretary and personal assistant for 25 years and who continues in this role today.

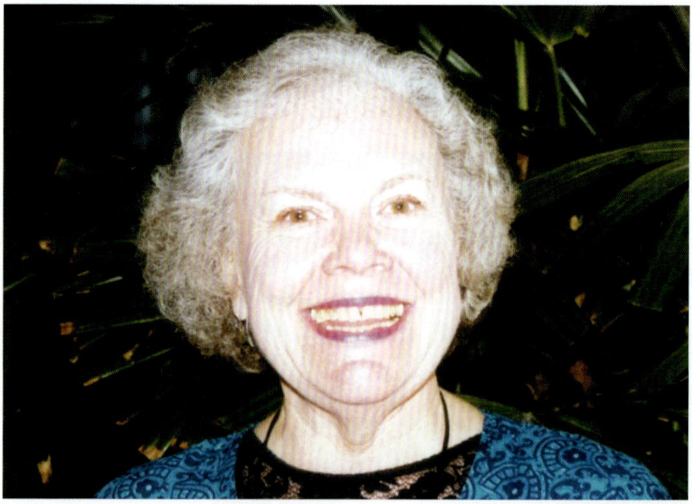

Ann Carlton, who provided accommodation and guidance to me and all the Institute faculty who taught in Dallas.

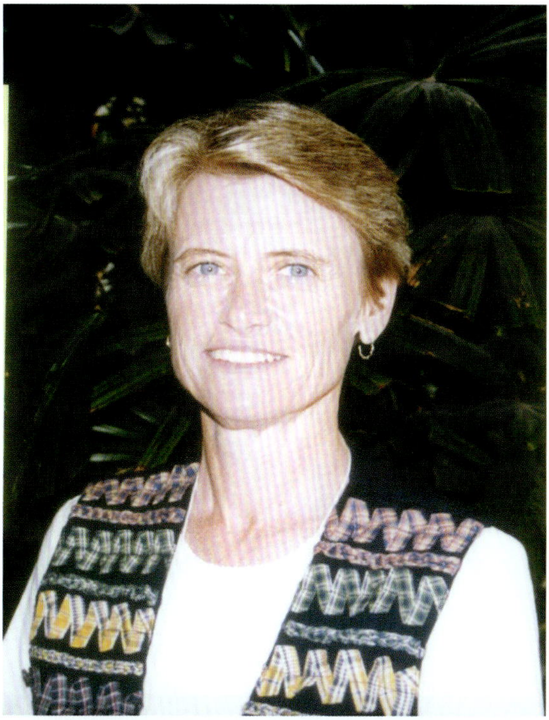

Kathy Hoyt, the physiotherapist who with Barbara Stone set MDT in motion and to this day is indispensable in the Institute's affairs.

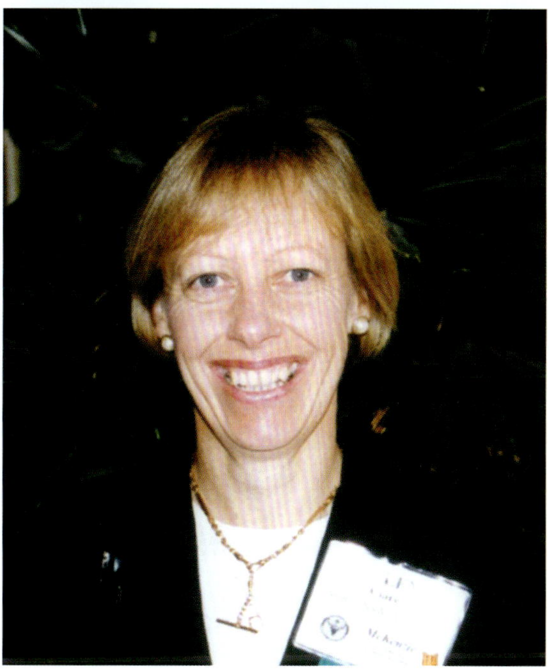

Dr Helen Clare, in her capacity of Director of Education, is the architect of the McKenzie Institute International education programme and the author of several important research projects.

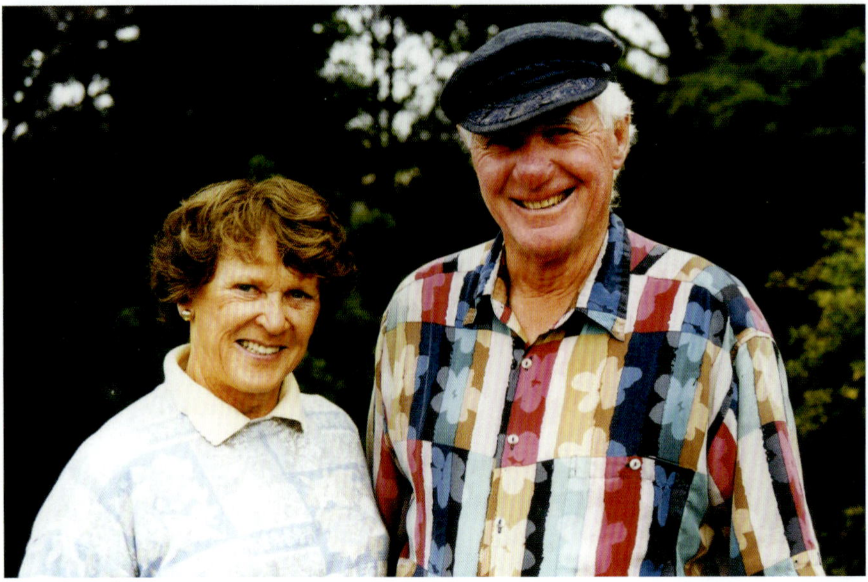

With Joy at End Farm, 1998.

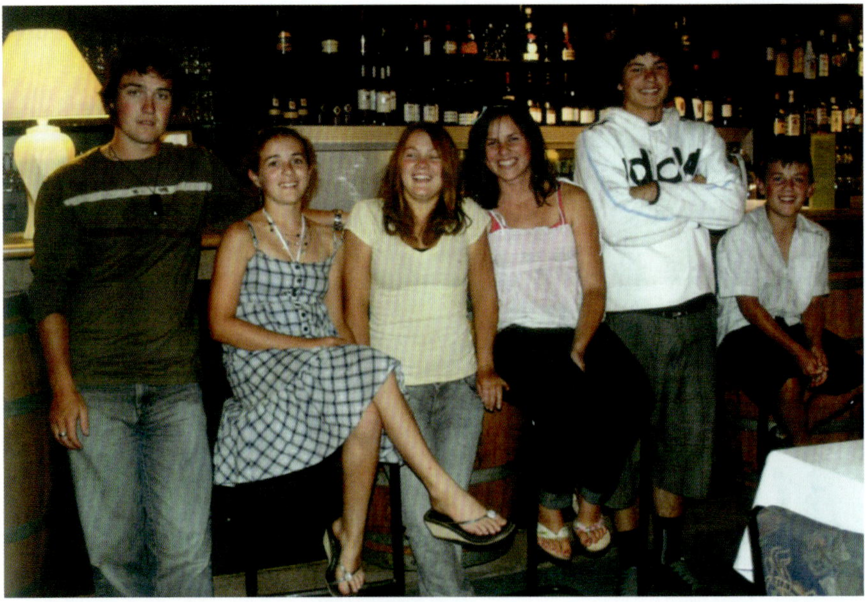

Our six grandchildren: Simon, Jessica, Melanie, Tamar, Cahn and Stuart, 2007.

and had no real intention of seeking the truth and that he suspected my real intention was to undermine and split the Association's membership.

Over five or so years with *Sundance* I had become a confident sailor and now decided it would be fun to enter a race to be held in conjunction with the British Commonwealth Games in January 1974. The start was in Auckland and it was scheduled to finish in Lyttelton, near Christchurch, where the Games proper were to be held. This would require *Sundance* to be fitted to meet the stringent safety rules governing such races. Also, of course, she would have to be sailed from Wellington to Auckland, a distance of some 400 nautical miles, where the race was to commence. The prospect appealed to me greatly and the rest of the family were keen too. David, at 14 years of age, was very useful and loved the boat and sailing.

Thus, with sailing friend Ron Cooke as first mate, we set sail for Auckland up the east coast at the beginning of the school summer holidays. The four days spent in a northeast gale, in which we had Castlepoint lighthouse in view every night, did not make for a good start. We were constantly buffeted by waves and wind and could make little headway. Every evening when it became dark, someone would ask if the light was still in sight. Every time I would have to admit that it was. During almost all of this time Joy and the children were lying below and were not at all happy.

Finally, on the evening of the fourth day, the wind changed direction and *Sundance* took off at good speed in the right direction. The next morning the family finally appeared on deck and were very excited to see a Royal Albatross was following close behind. The giant bird was paddling as fast as the yacht, which had slowed in the now light breeze. The albatross was just one of the many wonderful memories of that trip. He followed *Sundance* for four days. Travelling north the sea was obviously becoming warmer and one fine afternoon we were surrounded by a very large pod of whales travelling in the same direction. At first I was somewhat alarmed. There were whales in all directions as far as the eye could see, and many were much longer than the ketch. What would happen if one surfaced beneath us? There was nothing I could do except shut off the cabin entries to prevent water entering and flooding below were we to be tipped on our side. We just watched as we sailed in a light wind, with a flat sea, in company of this enormous armada that was very slowly overtaking us.

The next day, still in perfect conditions with a light wind, we witnessed a most strange motion of the sea. Knowing that we were about 50 miles from land, it was very odd to see turbulence in the water that resembled light surf against a sandy shore. We were about five or six hundred yards away, and heading towards this apparently stationary wave. As we moved closer the water behind the wave seemed about two feet higher than the level on which we were sailing, and as we sailed over it we could clearly see the difference in levels. I have since asked many other boaties if they have seen this phenomenon. No one has offered a credible explanation.

A few days after this, when we were motoring because of the lack of wind, one of the children noticed a large fish was jumping out of the water, and seemed to have been hooked on the fishing line that we had trailed behind the yacht since leaving Wellington. Ron, at the helm at the time, stopped the motor while I tried to reel the fish in. It was a losing battle as the fish had taken much line that the reel was almost empty. Ron and I jumped into the dinghy with the rod just as the fish again leaped out of the water. It was visible for just a moment, but long enough for us to see that we had hooked a swordfish! David turned the motor on and followed at a safe distance as the swordfish towed us in our little dinghy around the Bay of Plenty on the east coast of the island. Finally, after 30 or 40 minutes, we had the swordfish on deck – and fresh fish to last us a very long time. An expert in these matters later told us, from the photographs taken, that it was a very rare swordfish called a Broadbill and that we should have tried to bring it ashore rather than cut it up for steaks.

All this time we were travelling northwards and had not seen land for four of five days. That seemed rather strange as I had calculated that we should be just 10 or 15 miles off the coast, about 100 miles before the turn in towards Auckland. That day I had noted several jet streams from aircraft flying high above. I knew that the only international airport was at Auckland so why were they heading so far to our left. I suddenly began wondering where the hell we were. Prudence suggested turn hard left. Irrespective of a specific destination, west would take us somewhere on the east coast.

Forty-eight hours later we berthed in Whitianga in Mercury Bay on the Coromandel Peninsula, two to three days' sailing short of Auckland. We had a long conversation with the local policeman, who thought *Sundance* was just what he had always wanted. We stocked up with provisions and, now knowing where we were, set sail for Kawau Island which had been recommended as a safe anchorage.

We were almost at the island when a launch came up beside us, and having seen the name on the stern called out, 'Hey *Sundance*, don't you know you are hopelessly lost? Turn on the National News at five o'clock and you will hear that you're missing.' We could not believe this – who would have advised we were lost? We worked it out fairly quickly. We had a friend being married in Auckland, and before leaving Wellington we had casually mentioned that if we got to Auckland in time we would be at the wedding. We hadn't made it of course, and one of the party called the Police. Evidently a coastal police watch had been in force for five days but that message had not got to Whitianga, where the gendarme who thought our boat was just what he wanted was asleep at the time!

We made front-page news in the evening papers after reporting that we were having a nice holiday on Kawau Island. I had words with my friend, who though meaning well, had failed to realize that yachting is not an exact science and blew the whistle.

We arrived in Auckland a few days before the race was due to start. There were many things to do to ready ourselves for the race. On the start line we were last away. At the finish we were still last!

By 1975, four years after the Monaco meeting had sparked some interest but without greatly advancing acceptance and understanding of the method, I had essentially accepted that the difficulties were just too great. I discussed my financial situation with Peter Lawson, my accountant, who advised that the only way professional people could ever comfortably retire was to have an investment that would grow in value, with benefits derived from tax deductions on earnings. As a result of this discussion Joy and I decided that we would buy a 56-acre property in the seaside village of Waikanae, an hour north of Wellington, build a family home for our boys (Jan was now keen to be independent), raise some animals and grow our vegetables. We really wanted a quiet lifestyle that we could enjoy after years of hard work and the disappointment of the failure to achieve real recognition of the treatment methods I so believed in.

The Waikanae house site was on the top of a sand dune, 100 feet above sea level and 500 yards back from the sea itself. It had a commanding view of the coast, with the South Island visible across Cook Strait on clear days. One of my patients, a demolition manager, arranged for 30,000 old bricks from the demolition of the original Wellington Hospital kitchen to be dumped at the site, the deal being that I would take everything that came with the bricks, including roofing iron, spouting, smashed doors, windows, window frames, glass, broken paving, tiles and flooring. We spent weeks clearing all the junk and then hired a bulldozer to excavate an enormous hole into which the unwanted material was pushed and buried.

Before construction could start, the bricks had to be cleaned of the old mortar. At weekends Joy, the three boys, now in their teens, and I would clean and stack bricks around the site – an enormous job, but we had a mission. The house was built using about half of the old bricks, many of which were well weathered. Some of them had the convicts' arrow and a few showed thumb and finger prints identifying the manual origin of their manufacture. In the late 19th century, convicts laboured in the brickworks in Wellington and bricks made there carried the arrow imprint.

When completed, the house looked as though it had stood for decades. We moved into our new home on End Farm the following year, and I began building brick walls around the contours of the sand dunes on which the house was constructed. Tennis elbow and calloused hands were a minor consequence of this manual labour that would take about seven years to complete.

Jan now shared a flat in Wellington with friends. David, who had recently completed an apprenticeship at an Agriculture College, took on the management of a chicken farm, and Alistair and Andrew continued school in Waikanae. We acquired a delightful West Highland White Terrier – Rosie – now that we were settled on the farm. Joy and I devoted a lot of our time to developing the landscape and garden. I set about planting pine and eucalyptus trees over much of the property. There were large areas covered in fallen trees that had to be cleared before there could be new planting. We had a chicken coop which provided a constant supply of fresh eggs and we had an aviary with racing pigeons and doves.

To help clear some of the fallen trees and scrub on the farm we purchased an old Ferguson tractor, 1950s vintage. The gears and foot brake were well worn and not always reliable. I used to tie tree stumps to it and pull them into a heap to burn. On one occasion I was returning to the top of a hill for the next log when I noticed that a large branch was wedged under the front wheels. I stopped the tractor and attempted to pull the branch out from under the tractor frame. It would not budge at first but by working it back and forth it was beginning to loosen. I felt a slight twinge of pain in my back but it was not enough to stop my efforts. With a final heave the branch came free but that last pull caused such severe pain that I fell to the ground. I attempted to stand but the pain was extreme and I though it best to stay put for a while until it subsided. I then heard a slight sound coming from the tractor and looked up to find it slowly rolling back towards me. The branch had obviously held the tractor in place and removing it had set it in motion. I tried to roll away from its path but could not. Then it occurred to me to try my own prescription. I pushed myself into extension two or three times and looked again at the tractor. It was much closer. A few more push-ups and in panic I crawled out of the path of the one-ton monster which then rapidly gathered pace until it came to rest at the bottom of the slope. So *my* first episode of back pain was short-lived and I was pain free in 24 hours.

Joy was determined to grow our vegetables and spin and weave wool. Her woollen sweaters became much sought after and are worn by friends and family to this day. We were settling into a comfortable existence on End Farm.

CHAPTER 9

THE USA

I was 45 years old now and I still travelled into the clinic in Wellington every day. Colin Davies had left the clinic and was replaced by Tom Burgi, who was from Switzerland and fluent in German. I had also established a smaller clinic in Waikanae, hoping I might eventually work there for two or three days a week, which would be enough to 'keep the wolf from the door' so to speak.

Unbeknown to me, at about this time a New Zealand physiotherapist, Ace Neame, one of the first physiotherapists to recognize the value of MDT, was demonstrating to participants at a conference in the Canary Islands what he had seen me do with the patient on the film shown in Monte Carlo some five or six years earlier. Alice McCleary, a physical therapist from the United States, observed Neame's demonstration of my correction of acute lumbar scoliosis. Upon her return home she reported to her colleagues what this McKenzie fellow from someplace down under could do with difficult patients, and I soon received an invitation from two physical therapists, Kathy Hoyt and Barbara Stone, working at a large rehabilitation hospital in Los Angeles. They wanted me to visit and demonstrate my approach at the famous Rancho Los Amigos National Rehabilitation Center. I could hardly believe the letter in my hand as I had waited for an opportunity like this for so long. Perhaps this would make something really happen.

On that first trip to Los Angeles in 1977 I learned from Barbara and Kathy that the chief orthopaedic surgeon at Rancho Los Amigos was Dr Vert Mooney. He was very supportive of physiotherapy and also depended on physiotherapists' skills. Mooney was very prominent in hospital and professional circles. He was later to become President of the American Orthopaedic Association. After learning of my demonstration on extremely difficult patients, Mooney became very enthusiastic about the system in spite of it appearing to be diametrically opposite to everything being advised in the international scientific literature.

I had directed the course organizers to provide their most difficult patients for my presentation. I did four days of demonstration and explanation of the theory at Rancho Los Amigos. I relied mainly on my preferred method – of treating patients in front of other clinicians. I wanted to demonstrate with the most difficult patients they had, as effective treatment of these would impress observers most. What I did not know was how seriously disabled some patients in this American rehabilitation hospital were. The first patient I saw had had seven operations on his back. I was unsuccessful in treating him and equally unsuccessful with the second, who had had five operations. I fared no better with the third and my dismay was considerable. There happened to be a therapist in the audience observing me who had longstanding back problems and who volunteered on the spot to be treated in front of the group. Fortunately for me she responded so well over the four days that the observers felt that my approach ought to be given further consideration.

However, I had an overwhelming feeling that I was blowing this chance that I had put so much store by. I knew that one success out of 10 or 12 would not convince anyone of the value of my approach. Joy and Jan, our daughter, had accompanied me on this first exciting trip and were waiting for me in the motel room. I called for a large gin and tonic and told them I couldn't fix Americans and just wanted to go home.

Surprisingly though, the one successful patient had convinced Mooney of the value of my method and this was to prove the big break I needed. Mooney was so influential he could apparently make almost anything happen – and it did. To this day his support has been critical to my progress. Thanks to this very moderate success and the somewhat equivocal successes with the very complicated cases seen on the first visit to Los Angeles, I was invited back. On my second visit to Rancho Los Amigos Hospital, the following year, I was given patients who had more routine back problems that had not been complicated by surgery. I was able to demonstrate over a four-day period that I could make a huge difference to these patients, and I was able to improve the condition of some who had had persisting or recurring problems for years.

There was general surprise amongst the health professionals who observed my demonstrations that I was confidently able to determine the groups who would respond quickly, those who would respond more slowly, and those who would not respond. Another benefit was becoming increasingly apparent; the system was exposing an important advance in diagnosis. There were consistent response patterns amongst those who would benefit and now I was aware that any untypical adverse response to initial treatment often indicated a more serious condition was present. Back pain is not always uncomplicated and mechanical. Rather than providing treatment that I knew had no hope of success, I immediately referred those patients who did not respond to the appropriate specialist.

I was booked for further four-day courses in Los Angeles, San Francisco and Pittsburgh. The word was spreading and I was elated. There were 40–50 healthcare professionals in each group and the enthusiasm was infectious. It seemed that no one previously had ever taken live, unscreened patients and treated them in front of a group of professionals. I knew that in the average community I could demonstrate a 70 per cent success rate in the four days of the education seminars. This powerful teaching method was unique and the clinicians in the United States appreciated it immediately. At each course usually three or four people asked me if I would come to their hospital, and by the end of the tour in 1978, I had a dozen invitations for the coming year.

Of course not everyone was enthusiastic. Some clinicians who had become accustomed to being the local expert in treating back pain resented me and my intrusion on their patch. There were always one or two such people attending my courses and I began to identify them on the first morning of the first day. Instead of asking questions to clarify a misunderstanding or some other point, they would try to test the depth of my scientific knowledge, I suppose to cast doubt on my competence. I quickly learned how to deal with this hazardous aspect of lecturing. With the same questions arising everywhere I went, I developed somewhat evasive stock answers. 'There is insufficient supportive evidence to validate that research,' or, 'The jury is still out on that one', were two of the best, and both were very true at that time.

The standard treatment of low back pain in North America in the middle of last century had partially been set by a surgeon from Vancouver named Harry Fahrni. Fahrni was one of the first authorities to advocate flexion (bending forward) for treatment of low back pain. He based his philosophy on the grounds that in many cultures people sat on their haunches with the lower back flexed. This he claimed was the reason that North American Indians and people from tribes in Africa rarely suffered from back pain. He failed to recognize, however, that these people would rarely consult a European doctor, so the incidence of back pain in these populations was not included in the medical literature. His rationale nevertheless rapidly spread throughout North America, so it was not surprising that I was greeted with scepticism when I arrived in Vancouver to educate and demonstrate that exactly the opposite movements would improve over 70 per cent of low back pain patients.

On the morning of the first day two local therapists, who were the gurus of back pain treatment in the city, John Oldham and Chris Fowler, subjected me to the usual questions, testing my knowledge of the literature and challenging the theory. It so happened that the professor of history at Vancouver University was a patient on my first course. He had been treated for two or three months with no improvement by a local therapist who was also attending my presentation. After examining him and determining his pain was immediately treatable, I advised him to carry out the routine exercises that would resolve his problem. He returned the next day impressed with the results and by the third day of the course he was almost pain free. He said to me, "You know Mr McKenzie, your exercises are diametrically opposite to the ones I have been doing for three months. How do you explain that?" I replied diplomatically that as the exercises he had been doing had not helped, it was time to change them. He smiled and said in front of the whole group, "You don't fool me – they screwed up, didn't they?" He was completely better just a few days later.

At one course in Los Angeles I overheard two course participants in conversation. "What happens if he makes a mistake?" The implications of 'a mistake' had never entered my head. I hadn't considered the possibility of being sued if anything went wrong in the USA. On my next teaching tour I made sure, at great expense, that I was insured for any eventuality.

At last I had taken real steps on this long-awaited journey of sharing my knowledge. Scientists are generally very sceptical of any claim of a new cure, but every small step forward was now good enough for me. Scientists could be put aside; it was the clinicians I was relying on to prove my method. In the United States, those who found my demonstrations convincing went out and told others about the method, and so it went on. It was word of mouth to a large degree.

Some of the "early birds" were enormously supportive of me then and continued to play key roles in the development of the now-named "McKenzie Method". Dr Arthur White, an orthopaedic surgeon from San Francisco, became interested in the method and contributed a foreword to my first textbook. Vert Mooney became Professor of Orthopaedics in Dallas, Texas after leaving Rancho Los Amigos Hospital. He is one of the most prolific researchers in the field of spinal pain in the United States. He was president of the American Orthopaedic Association and the International Society for the Study of the Lumbar Spine. I owe so much to him for his support. Vert put me on the map!

Another of the key figures involved was Dr Ron Donelson, an orthopaedic surgeon from Syracuse. Ron was introduced to the method after his physical therapist Greg Silva attended my first course in Pittsburgh in 1978. As a surgeon, Ron was able to influence other medical specialists and promote my system in the US. Dan Kelley, from St Louis, was among the first group of clinicians to learn the method when studying at Kaiser Permanente Orthopaedic Clinic Residency Program in Hayward near San Francisco where I was guest lecturer in 1979. Studying with Dan at Kaiser was Kathy Hoyt. She was one of the two therapists in Los Angeles who had first invited me to visit. Her wisdom and intellect are unique in any company. Whereas I tend to make decisions on the spur of the moment, Kathy would in an instant foresee all possible consequences and potential pitfalls and evaluate them before making any decision. She became a very important ally in my cause.

On the home front Glen Pendergrast replaced Tom Burgi in the clinic in 1977. Glen began just as I was about to leave for an overseas meeting. After only two or three weeks' experience with processes that were new to him, Glen was left to sort things out as best he could. I did wonder if I would have any patients left on my return, but remarkably, he carefully read through the patient records and worked out how the system was applied. When I returned he was clearly very proficient in delivering effective treatment and I was both relieved and impressed.

On my 1977 visit to the US I presented three courses, in 1978 another 16, and 24 in 1979. As I travelled around the States I sometimes noticed that the same faces appeared at different courses in disparate parts of the country – in St Louis, Philadelphia, Los Angeles. Why were these people showing up again and again? It turned out to be nothing more sinister than that they wanted to learn more. Some said they observed slight differences with the treatment of a particular category of patient, which taught them variations of the principles. Amongst the repeaters, one gentleman stood out, resplendent in his US Air Force uniform and obviously of high rank. Ron Bybee attended some five or six of my courses and enthusiastically assured me he was learning more each time.

The momentum was enormous now – by 1980 I was booked through to the end of 1983. And then suddenly it all became too much to handle. Having waited so long for recognition of MDT, I now found I couldn't cope with the developments alone. But this was a wonderful problem to have after all this time.

From the ranks of my enthusiastic supporters I was able to recruit a superb team of teachers who knew the basic substance of the system almost as well as I did. They met regularly, especially when I was in the States, as I was more and more frequently, and eventually, in 1983, they made the decision to collectively organize courses and teach exactly the same material and format as I had done – under the umbrella of an institute.

The individuals I originally chose to start with came from the more populous states and cities in the United States. Kathy Hoyt and Barbara Stone were from Los Angeles, Dan Kelly from St Louis, Greg Silva from New York State, Hugh Murray from West Virginia, Wayne Rath from New Jersey, and Angelo di Maggio from Detroit. They were all committed to assisting in the education of the now very large group of healthcare professionals seeking to understand MDT. Their commitment and energy greatly accelerated the process of spreading the assessment and treatment protocols throughout the States.

In addition to my US-trained helpers, I decided to recruit some of my New Zealand physiotherapists to help with the load. This was an interesting period and a steep learning curve for me. I soon found that not all the enthusiastic helpers would stay the distance. Most, fortunately, were dedicated and motivated for all the right reasons, but a few took advantage of the popularity of MDT and went out on their own to teach independently. As well, problems arose when clinicians who had paid to learn the McKenzie Method were taught by independents who were not entirely competent and introduced incompatible variations.

In 1980 I was delighted to receive an invitation to demonstrate the system at Dallas General Hospital where Vert Mooney was now Professor of Orthopaedics. I called him on my arrival to advise where I was staying. Surprisingly, he said "I'll come right over". I waited at the entrance to the motel and then an old-model Volkswagen appeared from which Mooney emerged still wearing his white coat and stethoscope. He held out his hand and said, "Let's go and have a drink", which we did. The course was very successful. Dr Mooney sat through much of it and noted the polishing we had done to the presentation. I believe it strengthened his earlier recognition of the significance of MDT for rehabilitation of spine patients.

In 1983, the year the Institute was formed, Vert Mooney nominated me to be admitted to the International Society for the Study of the Lumbar Spine. At this time the Society was limited to 150 experts from around the world. I completed the application and submitted my books and materials and was accepted as a member of this very exclusive group. At that point I was only the second physiotherapist to be admitted, so I felt very privileged. Once again Vert Mooney helped me along the way.

Vert and I had become firm friends over the years and when together we would talk endlessly about the spine and all the possible mechanisms that could cause pain. Late one night, after a few glasses of whiskey, we discovered we were born one week apart in April 1931. I am the senior by one week. We then thought it incredible that although born on opposite sides of the planet one week apart we should share and be so involved in this common interest.

Not everyone was happy that I was receiving recognition by the Society. A local orthopaedic surgeon expressed his annoyance that an upstart physiotherapist who claimed that simple exercise could in many patients avoid the need for surgery could achieve the elevated status of membership. I could never have guessed that my admittance to the group would be so controversial. Many of the members were surgeons and were already firm believers in the old flexion-oriented treatment, which was the complete opposite to my method. They simply ignored my presence. This was of course distressing to me but I was buoyed up by the ever-increasing number of surgeons and therapists outside of the Society membership who were very impressed with what our trained therapists were able to do with so many of their patients. I had noticed that the composition of my audiences was slowly changing. More orthopaedic surgeons and other physicians were attending the seminars, most often because their therapists were achieving such impressive results with their patients that they came to see for themselves what it was all about.

I gained the impression that a number of the older Lumbar Spine Society members felt that my ideas represented just another of many faddish treatments for back pain that had no substance and that appeared and disappeared with monotonous regularity. Few took the time to understand the method and all I could do to teach Society members about my approach was to invite them individually to attend a course when I was giving one in their home area and to send their patients to be seen during the course. In this way more and more of them became acquainted with what I and other McKenzie-method-trained therapists were achieving.

Also in 1983 I was invited to speak in Chicago at the American Orthopaedic Association meeting. I could not help but recall the disastrous outcome of my first presentation to orthopaedic surgeons in New Zealand, but I felt confident now that the same thing would not happen again. I was given 20 minutes on the podium to describe my theory and treatment methods to the 2,000 surgeons present. I explained that if the patient was exercised at the extreme end of extension possible and the exercise was repeated frequently, the internal nucleus of the disc would be moved away from the nerve and the pain would reduce progressively. At the conclusion of my presentation a very prominent surgeon, John McCulloch, stood and asked why I continued to insist that the disc would move in this way. He and his fellow surgeons knew that it did not and in my claim I was certainly bringing my profession into disrepute.

I was speechless, having never before been confronted in such an aggressive manner. I could not think of a response that would mitigate the situation and humiliation overwhelmed me. Later, but too late, the answer I should have given was obvious – that if the disc does not move, why do surgeons have to operate to take out any displaced tissue? After that session, in the elevator on my way to my room, I encountered two or three others from the meeting. One questioned me: "Mr McKenzie, my understanding from your presentation is that you can take the pain from the leg in a surgical candidate and move it to the back so that surgery is no longer necessary. Is that correct?" When I replied "Yes, you could put it like that", he replied, "Some folk ain't gonna like that!" I couldn't appreciate the innuendo at the time. I left to return to New Zealand shortly afterwards, feeling a mix of anger, embarrassment and an enormous sense of futility, and vowing never to return to the United States. However, after a drink or two on the plane and after two or three more, the world seemed a little less hostile. My humiliation became resolution. I would go back – and I'd teach those bastards a lesson! And go back I did – many times.

After setting up the Institute in the USA, very quickly invitations were received from all over Europe and Australia to teach and demonstrate. The Institute was able to respond and then became established worldwide. Over the past four or five years Joy had sometimes travelled with me on short tours but often while I was away demonstrating and speaking she was left to care for the younger boys still living at home, and to take care of the farm and the garden. She had to hire and fire the farm helpers, who were not always very useful. I had often worried that I was absent so much both for Joy and for the children. I will forever regret the lost opportunities with the boys in their younger years – with my frequent and lengthy absences I missed out on some important experiences with them and I was not available to help in guiding them along the path to adulthood. Joy, though, was ever-present – a wise, wonderful, gentle mother, wife and person.

In November 1984 I held a ten-day meeting in New Zealand, at Waikanae, for hands-on training of American clinicians in the aspects of spinal manipulation I considered to be the most effective and reliable. I realized over time that if patients themselves could not apply sufficient force from the prescribed exercise, the clinician would sometimes need to add external pressure. Not all the physical therapists (as they were called in the United States) were trained in mobilization or manipulation, the procedures which could deliver that extra force. The meeting in New Zealand would provide an opportunity for them to learn the basics. Some of my colleagues assisted with the course and as well the Americans visited the clinics of Brian Mulligan, Paula van Wijmen, Mark Laslett and Ace Neame.

In 1986, following the meeting with the Americans in New Zealand, we realized that although the McKenzie Institute International had been inaugurated and was thriving in the USA, there was as yet no formal entity in New Zealand. Paula van Wijmen, Ace Neame, together with Rob Reid, Tom Burgi and I founded the McKenzie Institute New Zealand. Paula, Ace and Mark Laslett continued to participate as members of the International Institute faculty until the middle of the 1990s. Grant Watson, Greg Lynch and Graeme Nuttridge, who took over the responsibility of providing education internationally, followed them. Long-time member Celia Monk has been both president of the New Zealand Branch and has recently become a faculty member. Stuart Horton is attached to the Physiotherapy School at Otago University and has tutored the postgraduate students attending the Diploma Programme. Cheryl Hefford is currently tutoring for the University of Otago School of Physiotherapy Clinic at Victoria University in Wellington. All of the New Zealand faculty have in various ways contributed enormously to the growth of the Institute at home and internationally.

Those in the core US group were moving along with shaping the just-formed Institute and were working out precisely what should be taught over a four-day training session. They agreed immediately that all would teach the same material and present in a uniform manner, and also believed that seeing actual patients on the courses was a powerful teaching tool and it should continue. They committed to treating the patients exactly as I had treated them to protect the integrity of the method. This dedicated group played an enormously valuable role in establishing this early organization and standardizing the teaching methods. I don't know what I would have done without their ideas and support. They encouraged me greatly. For instance, Barbara Stone said to me on completion of a course in Los Angeles,

"Robin, you just don't know what you have done for physical therapy in the United States." I don't think I really was fully aware of the movement that was now well under way. Two years later I was made an Honorary Life Member of the American Physical Therapy Association and that honour brought this home to me.

And so finally, after years of frustration, I was involved almost full time in educating clinicians by treating patients before usually fascinated audiences. With the commitment of our team it was not long before the McKenzie exercises were known throughout the length and breadth of the United States. Newly trained therapists would return to their clinics and thereafter present physicians with patient improvement or cures they could not comprehend – they were unaccustomed to seeing such rapid changes.

CHAPTER 10

BOOKS AND BOATS

To ensure my patients had sufficient grasp of my instructions to continue self-treatment at home and at work, for some years I had provided them with the details in writing, with appropriate variations according to their individual problems. I described the exercises they were to do and how often to do them. I wrote down the restrictions on their activity during the recovery period and the sitting and standing postures. The pages of notes for each patient grew from five to eight to ten pages. I knew there was a better chance of them adhering to the rules if the instructions were in writing. If they exercised as instructed, the results were usually excellent. I told them that I could tell if they had not been doing the exercises and there was no way they could conceal that from me. I always, half jokingly, warned of the dire consequences of failing to comply. I was, though, becoming very tired of repeatedly writing out all these instructions for patients.

One day in 1979, some two years after my first teaching visit in the USA, an old friend from Wairarapa College, Hugh Price, appeared at my Wellington clinic. He was in great pain and bent over. He could not straighten up nor move because of the severity of the pain. It was a typical acute lumbar scoliosis identical to the patient on the film I had taken to Europe in 1968. Hugh had heard from others about what his old friend was doing with patients with back pain and decided to give me a try. He had experienced recurrent episodes of the same problem at least 25 times. It was so painful that many times he would be bedridden for more than a month. I was able to straighten him up and relieve his pain in a day. I gave him a set of notes and he went away very satisfied knowing that he could, to a large extent, manage his own treatment in the future. In fact, he had only one or two difficult episodes in the next ten years rather than the two or three recurrences per year that he had previously experienced.

Hugh owned a publishing company, Price Milburn, which mainly published children's books. On hearing about my writing chore he suggested that I should produce a book about what I was doing and include the instructions to the patients with my very busy clinic. I could not see how I would ever be able to find the time to do this and as well I was not confident about my writing ability. Perhaps in gratitude for what I had done for him, Hugh offered to write it up if I would explain it all to him in greater detail. So in 1979, armed with the Kelvin Chamber patient instruction notes, Hugh Price took off to Sydney for a week in isolation to write up the book on self-treatment.

On his return, I made a few corrections and additions to his manuscript and Hugh arranged for 2,000 copies to be printed. I was becoming concerned about how much all of this was going to cost me. The idea was that after enough books sold to cover the publisher's costs, the rest would be left to me to do with as I pleased. That way I would be able to supplement my income from the clinic in Wellington and the proceeds would be more generous than the basic royalty from a publisher.

The first edition of *Treat Your Own Back* (1980, New Zealand University Press/Price Milburn) was an immediate success. The books were advertised in local papers and sold very quickly. Another 10,000 copies were quickly printed and with the publishing costs covered, Hugh suggested that in future I arrange to print the book on my own. We decided to establish a publishing business for this purpose and after much thought I came up with the name Spinal Publications.

Spinal Publications printed a further 10,000 copies of the book in 1981. Joy and I were both over the moon with the success of the book. When I introduced *Treat Your Own Back* to the therapists I was teaching in the United States, they all wanted multiple copies to distribute to their patients, so yet another 10,000 copies were printed.

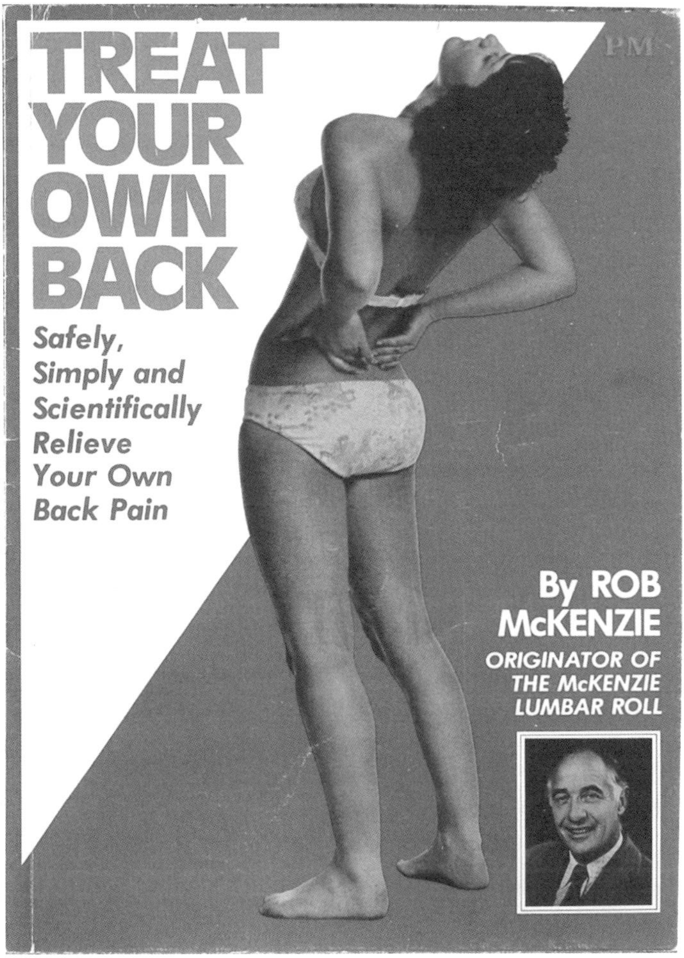

Treat Your Own Back. Cover of the first edition, 1980.

In the early days, once home in the evenings, Joy and I would open the small mountain of mail containing orders for the books. We would then spend the weekend packaging up the books on the dining room table and send them off to all parts of the world. We would go to the post office each week with several large boxes and many smaller packages to post overseas and soon the Waikanae post office complained that their weekly run of packages was overtaxing their two staff members. They asked if we could take them to Wellington where larger facilities could cope.

Demand had actually outgrown our ability to handle it. Someone had to be hired to manage the growing business and our daughter, Jan, in her mid-20s, was available and willing and agreed to take the job on, at least for a limited time. So in 1981 she joined the family publishing business.

With the immediate and ongoing success of *Treat Your Own Back* I realized that this extra income could in due course enable me to retire from practice. This became more obvious when, as time passed, I began to see that the self-help system was proving as effective for patients with neck problems as it had been for people with lower-back problems, and I decided to repeat the format for a new self-treatment book, *Treat Your Own Neck*, published in 1983. I would be ever grateful to Hugh Price for having provided the solution to my retirement worries and stimulating me to make self-treatment available on such a scale.

As sales increased it became necessary to develop some means to make the popular *Treat Your Own* series more readily available in the United States. Freighting books in large volumes from New Zealand was expensive and increased the costs to the reader. Shari Hanson Schroeder of OPTP, a company supplying physical therapy equipment, was suggested as a distributor for the books and also for the lumbar-roll supports that, as mentioned earlier, were essential for improving the back condition of many patients. Shari immediately recognized the need to provide MDT clinicians with the rolls and she organized their manufacture in the United States in 1982.

With the demand for teaching that was growing in America and the development of interest in Europe and Australia I knew that I would soon have to complete the textbook describing the essential elements of my method I had started in the late 1970s but that was still in skeleton form. Many clinicians in the United States had attended a course and taken notes but it was now clear that these were often insufficient and inaccurate. This led to many mistaken diagnoses and inappropriate treatments being delivered and it was obvious this had the potential to discredit the value of the McKenzie Method. There was therefore an urgent need to provide the teaching faculty of the

US Institute with the theory and procedures in written form. The European scene was developing too. My assistant in New Zealand, Paula van Wijmen, who had joined the clinic after Glen Pendergrast left in 1979, had been very helpful in a new edition of *Treat Your Own Back* and was now willing to organize this monograph for teaching.

I knew that I would be able to describe the theory and methods without much difficulty, but was concerned about the difficulties of presenting the theory itself. Would the theory be ridiculed? Would that lead to rejection of the whole because part was still conjecture? I worried for some time over these questions and then decided to include *almost* everything and to hell with the consequences. I decided not to include those elements that, although true according to my observations, were unbelievable to some. For instance, in carefully selected patients I could make the pain move from one side of the spine to the other, and then back again, but without witnessing it themselves, no scientist or researcher would believe that. I had already decided on the title, written the basic structure in draft form, and described the procedures for my first textbook, *The Lumbar Spine: Mechanical Diagnosis and Therapy.* This simple text, published in 1981, allowed clinicians to classify patients with low back pain and to provide appropriate treatment. To date between 40,000 and 50,000 of these books have been sold to healthcare professionals worldwide and it is clear that these clinicians are able to reproduce the results that I had claimed would eventuate if they followed the system faithfully.

In 1990, when I was still travelling to the USA regularly, I published a textbook describing my method for treating the remaining areas of the spine, *The Cervical and Thoracic Spine: Mechanical Diagnosis and Therapy.*

In the limited leisure time available we continued to have adventures on the sea with family and friends. Many memorable ones were those experienced on a converted pilot boat, *Manaia*, which we bought in 1987. *Manaia* was 73 feet long, weighed 20 tons and was powered by two Rolls Royce engines. When this boat was advertised for sale in

Whangarei, a town in the far north of New Zealand, I decided it was worthwhile travelling up to see if she would be suitable, but business commitments got in the way and I could not make the journey. In the meantime, unbeknown to me, *Manaia* was brought down to the Marlborough Sounds on trial for a prospective purchaser. One weekend we were sailing with friends in Queen Charlotte Sound and were struck by the sight of this fine looking vessel at anchor in one of the local bays. *Manaia* was still for sale and the price was going down. Her interior was in its original condition and was rather different from that of a cruising vessel. Realising that alterations would be expensive, I negotiated with the owners and a deal was struck. After the interior renovations *Manaia* could accommodate up to 12 guests and crew, had a complete galley and dining area and was a very seaworthy, go-anywhere vessel.

In 1991 we invited eight friends to join us in a cruise to the southernmost fjords in the south west corner of New Zealand. With four of my long-time sailing companions as crew I took *Manaia* from Picton at the head of the Marlborough Sounds and sailed for the fjords down the east coast. We had to negotiate a treacherous passage through Foveaux Strait between the bottom of the South Island and Stewart Island. The strait had a rather fearsome reputation, but on the day, *Manaia* passed through on a calm sea with no wind and we arrived in Dusky Sound four days after leaving. The following day, relieved that the journey so far was uneventful, we sailed north to Doubtful Sound where we were joined by our guests who had flown from Wellington. For the next eight weeks we travelled through the various sounds and the bays within, enjoying the spectacular scenery of this remote and unspoiled corner of the world.

In 1996, when I had to a large extent given up accepting invitations to teach and demonstrate overseas, we again took *Manaia* and friends on a long holiday. This time we travelled north into the Pacific visiting the various islands in the Tongan group and on the return voyage called at the Kermadec Islands. These were wonderful and well-earned leisure days for Joy and me.

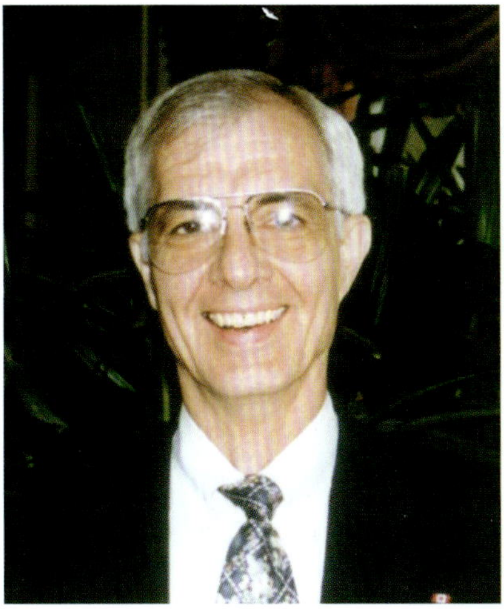

Ted Dreisinger has been a pillar of strength to both me personally and to the International Institute. With his dedication and perseverance the International MDT Research Foundation was successfully launched in 2008 to provide funds for research into MDT.

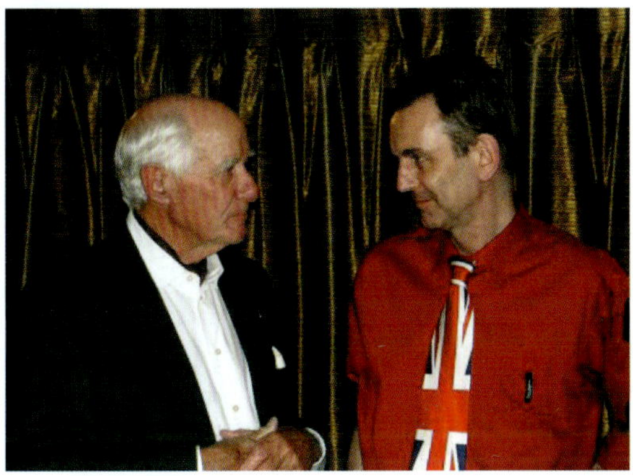

With Dr Stephen May, celebrating our co-authored text's publication.

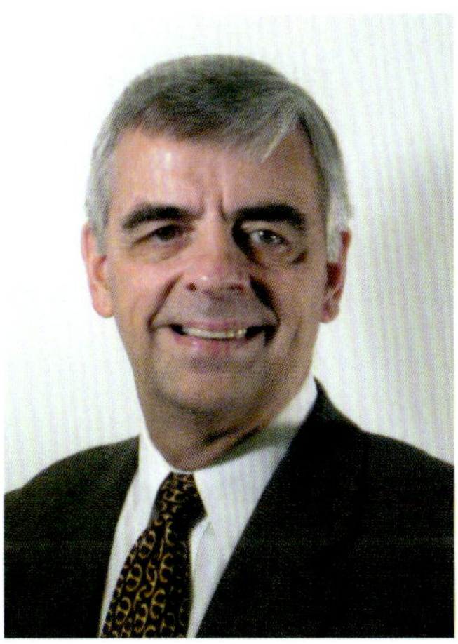

Ron Donelson has been a part of the Institute from the beginning. His contributions have been, and continue to be, of inestimable value to me to and the Institute. He is the author of Rapidly Reversible Low Back Pain, *an exposé of the biases of the scientific decision-makers.*

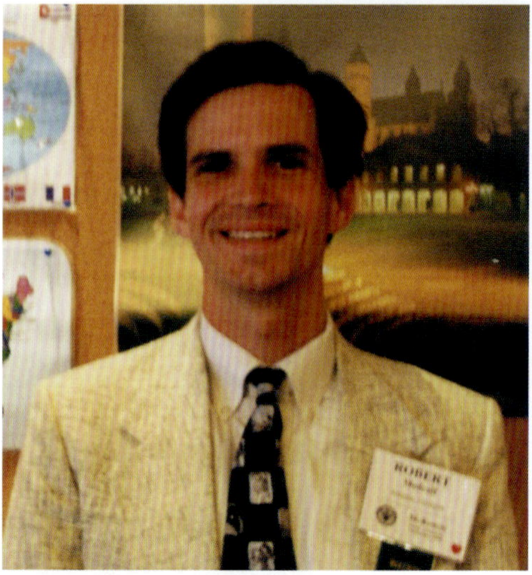

Robert Medcalf, my assistant on the first MDT course in Japan.

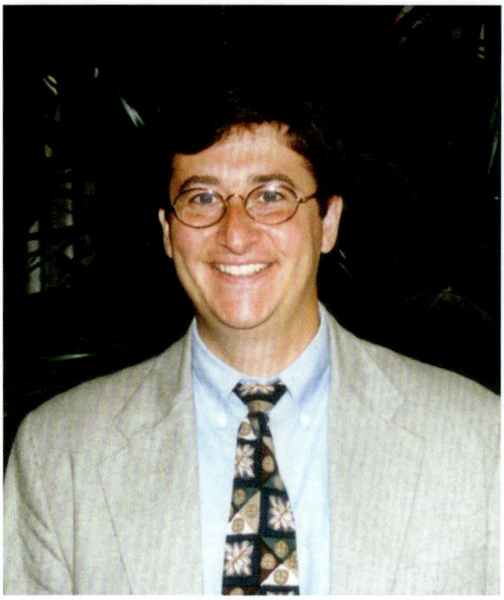

Dana Greene. Dana accompanied me to China to present the first demonstration of MDT to the medical profession there.

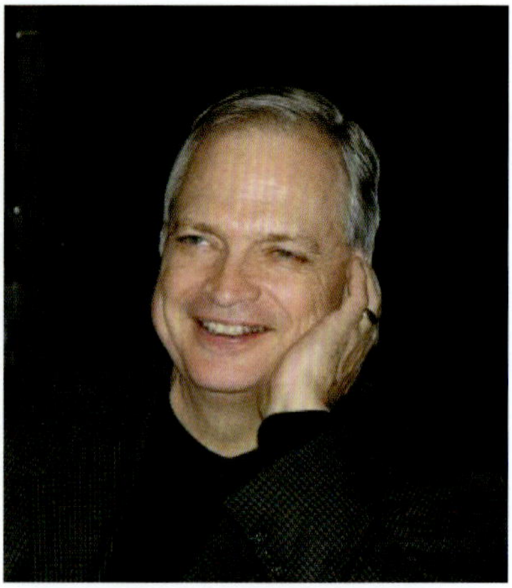

Dan Kelley, President of the Institute Board of Trustees.

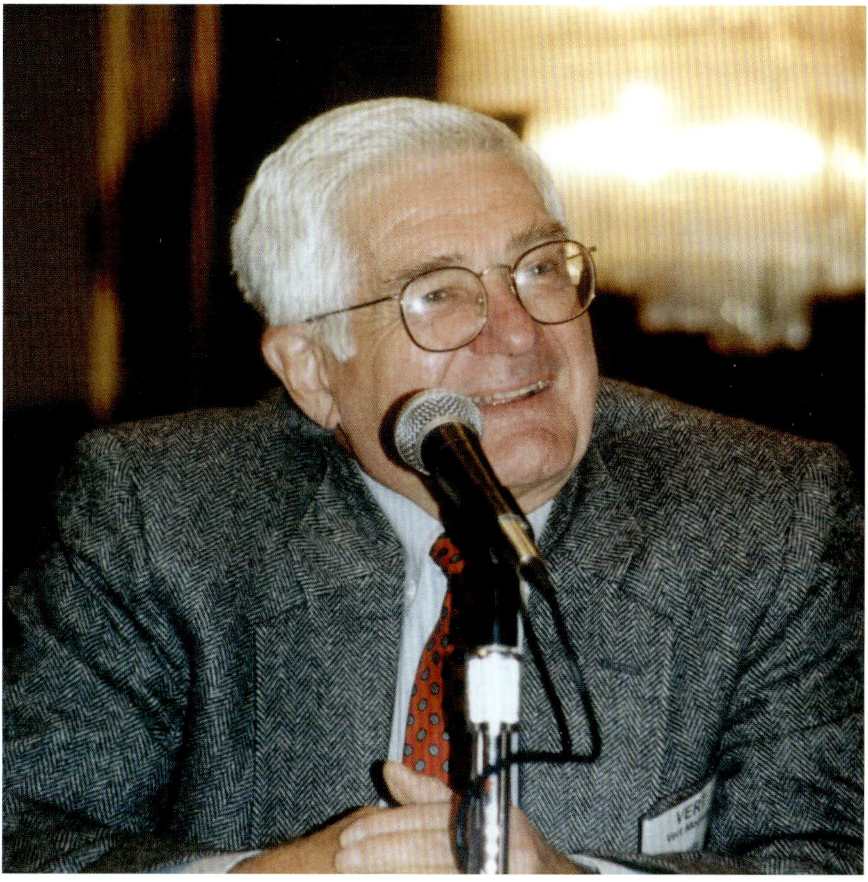

Vert Mooney, who made it all happen. Without his backing I would have retired to End Farm and MDT *would never have become recognized.*

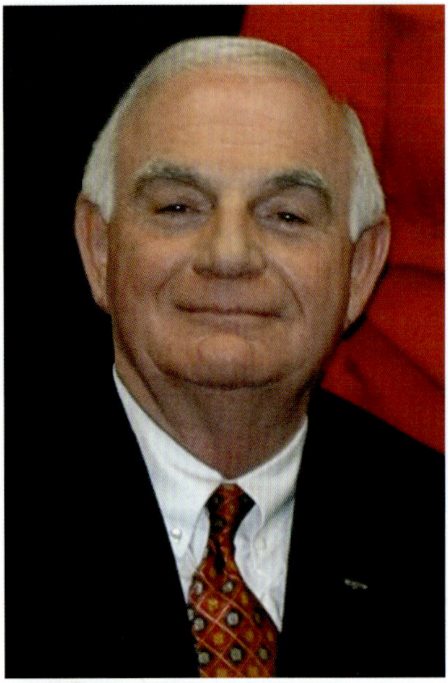

Ron Bybee, who has contributed greatly to this autobiography and been a huge supporter of the Institute over many years.

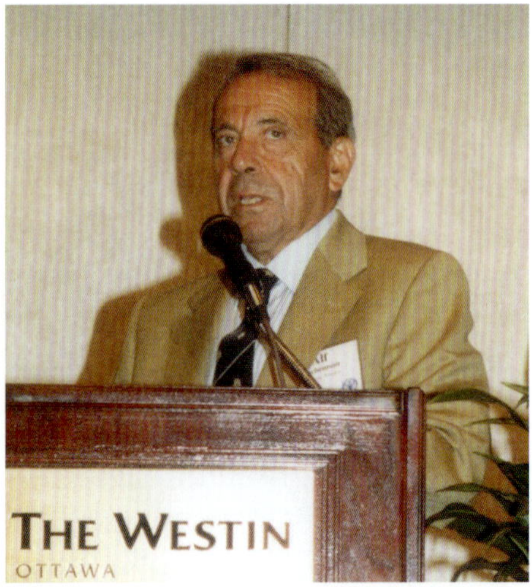

Alf Nachemson. A strong critic of orthopaedic surgeons and physiotherapists who operate unnecessarily or provide useless treatments. Prof Nachemson has spoken at many of our conferences and as time went by he warmed to the Institute's philosophies, finally acknowledging that we seemed to be providing something useful for patients. Praise indeed!

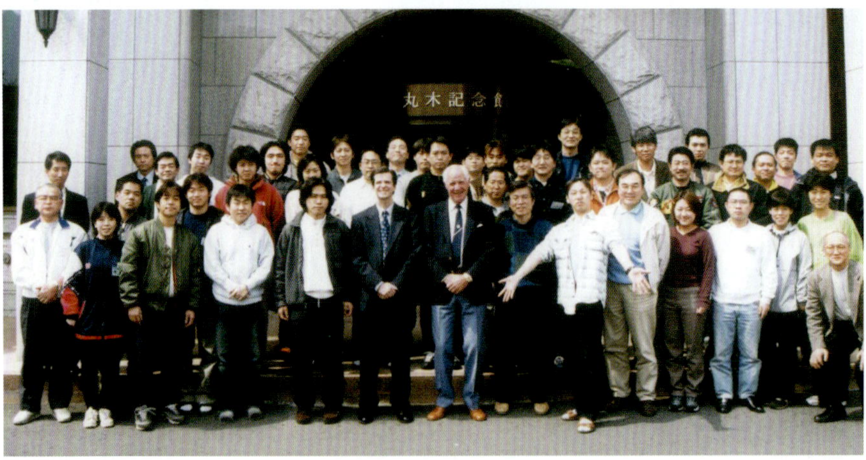

Robert Medcalf and myself at the first course in Japan, 2000.

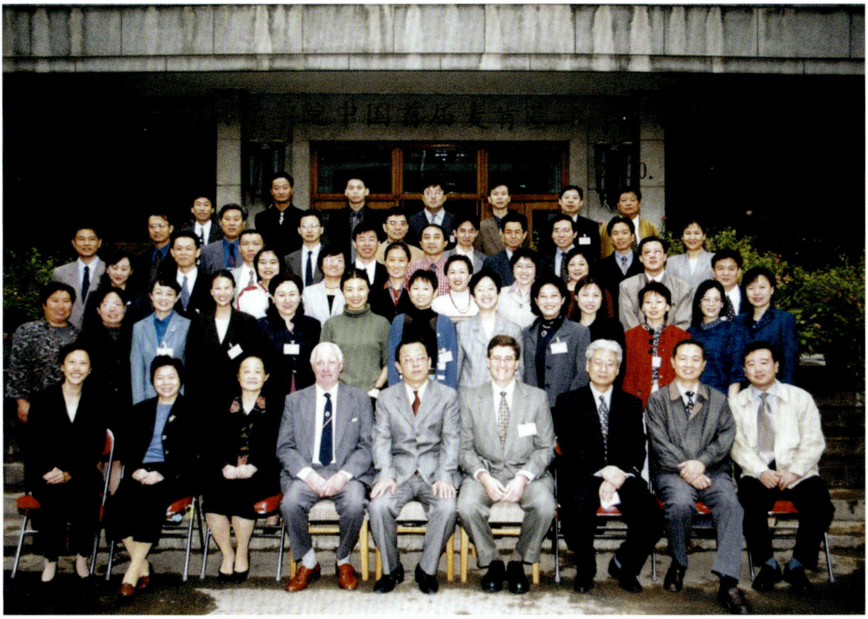

With the President of Beijing Hospital and Dana Greene (centre front row) at the first MDT course in China for medical practitioners, September 2000.

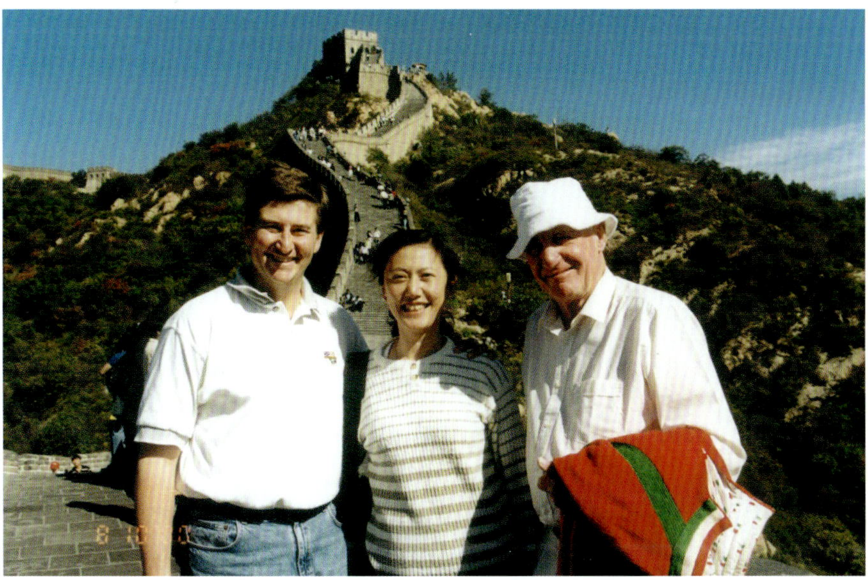

With Dana Greene and Dr Cynthia Gu at the Great Wall.

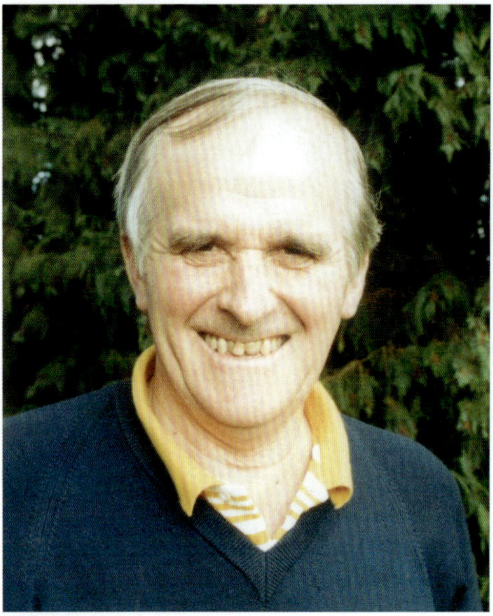

My dear friend from Army days, Warren Austad. He is now retired from medical practice and is the president of our Safari Golf Club.

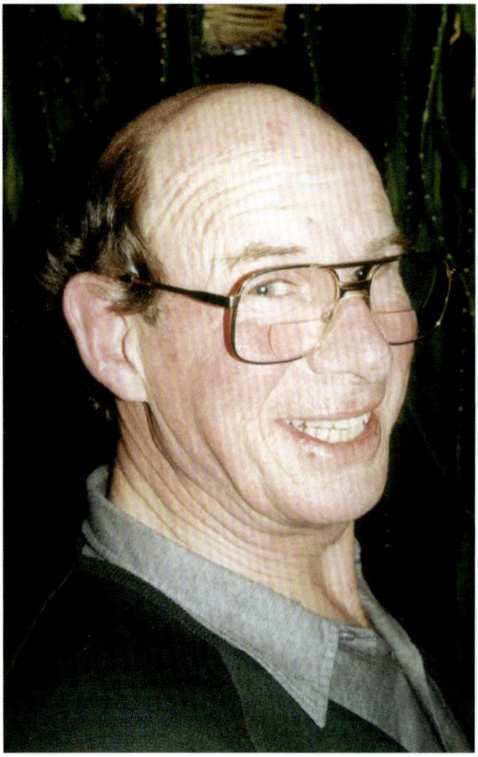

Graeme Law, another great and unforgettable friend from Army days. Sadly he passed away in 2003.

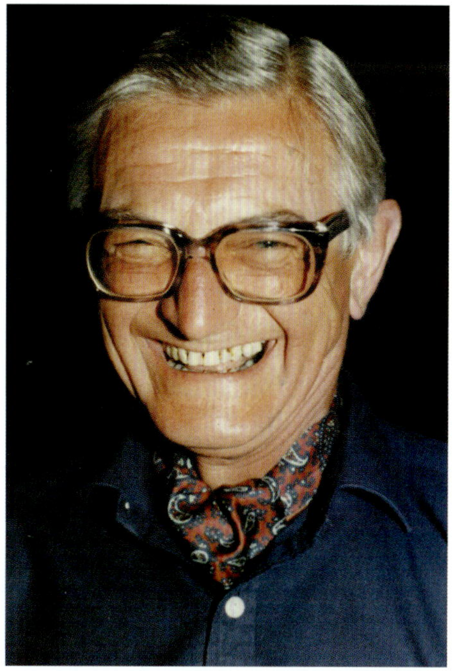

The late Dr David Wright, an old friend and founding member of the Safari Golf Club, who played a vital role in monitoring patients at the Institute Rehabilitation Centre in the early 1990s.

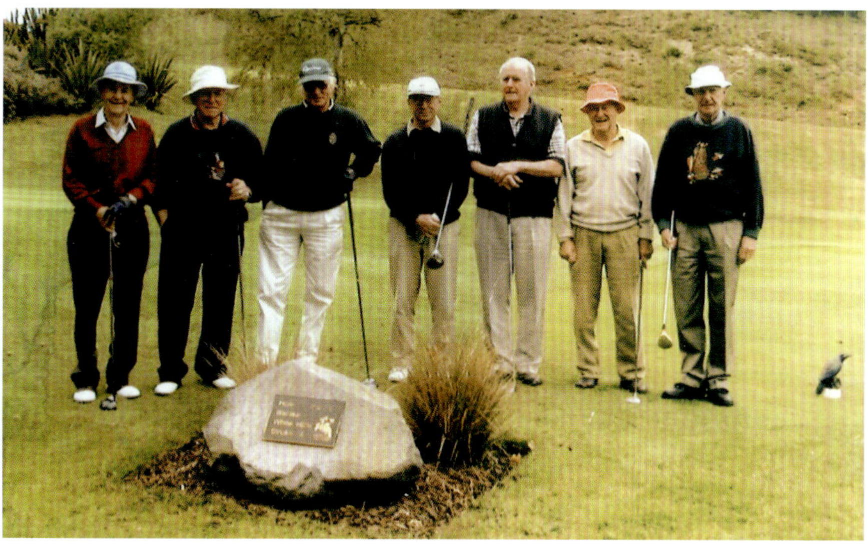

Members of the Safari Golf Club at Wairaki Golf Club, 2003. Bill Morris, Alan Harris, Charles Speight, Peter Hunter, Warren Austad, Bill Wiggins and me.

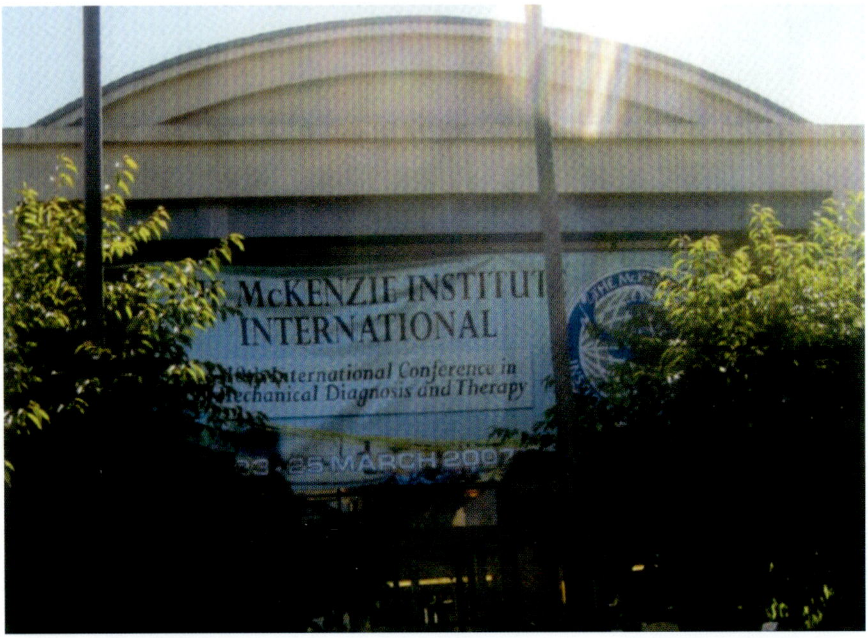

Millenium Hotel, Queenstown, the venue for the Institute's 10th International Conference, 2007.

I had concluded since the 1960s that the basic principles of MDT as it applies to the spine could be applied to the joints of the arms and legs, and indeed to the whole musculoskeletal system. I had been encouraged to record the details of the process many times but I was involved with so many aspects related to teaching methods and education of faculty within the Institute that the time necessary to produce another book was just not available. In 1998, I sought the help of Stephen May from the United Kingdom. He was one of the Institute's most senior figures and an expert on spine-related research and the physical therapy literature in general. Stephen agreed to collaborate on a book on methods for diagnosis and treatment of extremity joints and this resulted in our co-authoring *The Human Extremities: Mechanical Diagnosis and Therapy* in 2000. Soon to follow, also with very significant input from Stephen, were the second editions of *The Lumbar Spine: Mechanical Diagnosis and Therapy* (in 2003) and *Cervical and Thoracic Spine: Mechanical Diagnosis and Therapy* (in 2006). These had now grown to two volumes each. With Stephen's enormous contribution, especially his provision of a complete compendium of the scientific data supporting the McKenzie Method, these texts have become the gold standard for the non-surgical management of musculoskeletal disorders.

Also in 1998 Craig Cubey, a freelance journalist in California, approached me proposing that we rewrite the *Treat Your Own ...* books together. Cubey believed it would be advantageous to rewrite these especially for the American market, using American English. While I was not excited about the prospect, and unsure of Cubey's ability to influence US publishers, I agreed to assist in the writing of *Seven Steps to a Pain Free Life*, the title proposed by Cubey and the publisher. The book was by no means an instant hit, but was for a short time one of Amazon's top five.

CHAPTER 11

SIBERIA

In 1991 I was invited by the Russian Academy of Medical Sciences to introduce the McKenzie concepts and methods to Russia, initially through the Siberian branch of the Academy. After lengthy negotiations I set forth for Irkutsk, in Eastern Siberia, on 17 March 1993. I took the unusual step of keeping a diary of what was to prove a most memorable adventure.

I considered myself well travelled by now, and had experienced the complete spectrum of events, both pleasant and unpleasant, that might overtake one when regularly venturing abroad. Nothing could surprize me, or so I thought.

It was apparent at a very early stage in the journey that things weren't going according to plan. I was driving toward Wellington Airport when I remembered that my razor was recharging in the bathroom alongside my essential toilet bag. Having on various other trips had to purchase new electric razors for similar reasons, I called Joy and turned around to meet her as she rushed to my assistance one more time. Similar memory lapses with regard to wallets, passports etc. have honed her anticipation of such occurrences.

My luggage was booked right through to London without any problems, and I relaxed on an uneventful and pleasant flight through to Gatwick. A night in London, at the Excelsior Hotel, allowed me to catch up on sleep before my departure to Moscow the day after.

My flight from London to Moscow was leaving at 1.30 p.m., but I checked in with Aeroflot three hours before. My luggage was duly, and surprisingly, checked through to Irkutsk and I marvelled that such efficiency was possible, especially as I expected a long wait in Moscow. I boarded the plane at 1 p.m. and we took off shortly thereafter.

I was somewhat dismayed that no one on board seemed to understand or speak English. The Captain made an announcement on the audio system. At first I thought he was attempting to communicate in English but he was drowned out by the speaker system continuing to play a distorted version of "The Red Flag" that sounded like an old wind-up gramophone running out of steam.

It was difficult to communicate my requirements to the two hostesses and steward who were exclusively at my service. They continued to speak confidently in Russian but I quickly resorted to sign language. I was not at all embarrassed, for I was the sole occupant in this 40-seat first-class section.

Now came the matter of food. After much repeated gesturing on my part a salad arrived. It was a sorry sight – giving the impression of having been left out in the sun for several days and then doused in boiling oil. The chicken I ordered turned out to be fish. I contemplated the various strategies whereby I might exchange the old fish for the desired chicken, but the task of telling the stewardess that she had given me the wrong dish was just too onerous. I tackled it valiantly – it was almost inedible and left tough strings of fibre between my teeth. Suddenly the steward decided that I had had long enough to consume the fish dish, and removed it hastily, I think apologising in Russian, and replaced it with chicken. This, while not appetising in appearance, was satisfying enough. While I declined the vodka offered, I accepted the constant replenishing of my wine glass.

We landed in Moscow at 8 p.m. By now it was Friday evening and my flight to Irkutsk was not due to leave until 4.00 a.m. on Saturday morning, almost eight hours later. I waited with another 80 or so passengers at the luggage carousel. But an hour and a half later the original 80 had been replaced by another 200 passengers and my luggage had not appeared. I now assumed that it must somehow have gone all the way to Irkutsk. It would therefore not be necessary for me to clear it through the Customs as I had expected.

I passed through Immigration without any difficulties and was immediately set upon by six or seven taxi drivers, all of whom looked like ex-heavyweight boxers, with fists like the hind legs of lamb. There was a scramble to assist me with my hand luggage and camera and although I found myself shouting "Nyet, Nyet!" the harassment continued as I walked on. The first group of ex-boxers was simply replaced by a second and then a third wave.

There are only three notices in English at Moscow International Airport: "Customs Declaration", "Toilet" and "Information". No one in "Information" spoke English, even though Moscow International Airport is an official international tourist route. I started to consider the implications of this sinister circumstance, realizing how helpless I was.

Eventually I was found by the lady from In-Tourist Travel who did speak English, and who now told me that it was 105 kms, across or around Moscow, to the domestic terminal – Domodedovo Airport! The journey would be by taxi and the fare US$50. I did wonder how my luggage would, independently of me, have reached that distant airport and gone on to Irkutsk.

I accepted the inevitable and had a most fascinating taxi ride across Moscow at 11 p.m., for that is how long it took to get this far. The In-Tourist lady had further informed me before I departed that there was no such flight as Aeroflot 127 leaving at the time advised by my travel agent. I was though expected on another flight that fortunately was delayed and she thought I would likely make it on time.

On arrival at Domodedovo I was told by another In-Tourist helper that not only had the flight originally advised by my agent been terminated, but it did not go through Irkutsk. But my luggage could well have gone to wherever it was that that particular flight did now go to. This caused me no small amount of consternation. Further, she told me that the flight that I had been transferred to, Flight 121 to Irkutsk, was now running several hours later still. I would now be leaving at 7 a.m.

When you have travelled 13,000 miles from New Zealand to Russia and you know you have no bed for the night, and it is now midnight and that you have to check in at six in the morning, the fuse, already shortened by continuous stress, is very short. All the seats in this very very dirty airport are full of very very dirty people. The smell is ghastly and I am convinced that I have probably made the biggest mistake of my life. I did have one thing to be thankful for, that Joy had wisely decided not to come. This was not the sort of misery I would want to share with her. I was seriously wondering if I could somehow catch a plane back to London and then home, but the thought of another cab drive in the early hours of the morning to an airport which was probably closed shut down this fantasy.

I was so tired and stressed – perhaps I should have called up the fortitude of my Scottish ancestors who arrived in hostile New Zealand as settlers in 1850. I should be counting my blessings, and even enjoying the challenges of travel in modern-day Russia. A chart on the wall, to my amazement, showed me that this vast country occupied 11 time zones.

Departure time was finally approaching and I determined to seek the correct waiting lounge in good time. The In-Tourist desk was now closed. After searching for half an hour, all the time waving my ticket, a woman directed me to a door that opened onto the tarmac. It was freezing and windy outside. I closed the door, which seemed to irritate the lady, who then insisted volubly that I take my hand luggage and myself outside. I did and the door was shut behind me. Amazingly, a bus appeared and the driver beckoned. Steeling myself for another stressful mystery experience and casting all caution aside, I jumped into the bus, in which I was the sole occupant. It wound its way around a very dark airport for 15 minutes and eventually arrived at a departure lounge. I so hoped it was the right one.

I entered and found longed-for warmth as well as the most motley and evil-looking and smelling band of peasants I have ever seen. Surrounded by their meagre belongings, they were clothed in a variety of old ragged clothing, worn leather jackets, carrying sack-cloth bags with rough cord for shoulder straps or ancient leather bags and in shades of Genghis Khan, I could see that some had knives in sheaths strapped to their belts. The Mongolian and Asiatic features of peoples in this area is easily understood when you locate Irkutsk on the map of Siberia. I was fascinated to see groups of these people unroll their mats and undertake their prayers as the day dawned. They, at least, knew where East was.

In disbelief, I suddenly realized I was hearing English spoken – a party of seven Canadian miners, and going to Irkutsk! I tagged along behind them, determined to stay close to people who could understand my plight if anything worse befell me. My sense of wellbeing increased immeasurably. After carefully positioning myself to catch any stray snippets of information to assist my passage I learned that the plane would stop twice on the journey for refuelling. I wondered what sort of a plane requires refuelling twice in a seven-and-a-half-hour flight.

I passed the remainder of an extremely uncomfortable night eavesdropping on the Canadians, alternately sitting and standing, and walking up and down stairs to try to keep warm. The heating system had either failed or been turned off many hours earlier.

How the Canadians knew our flight had been called I could not determine, but when they moved, I moved. I could now see that Flight 121 to Irkutsk was boarding because the lights on the Departures board were flashing, although the lighting in the departure lounge had itself been flickering from time to time. Very little seemed certain.

With a boarding pass but no seat number, I followed the Canadians to the plane. I immediately noted on moving through the plane that the seating would not provide good lumbar support, but doubted there would be any value in advising Aeroflot of this. My seat choice was a poor one – as I sat down it reclined fully and nothing I tried would fix it in the upright position. The hostess did not seem to care and at this point I wondered if maintenance of the engines had been similarly neglected. I was resigned to my fate – certainly beyond believing anybody would provide any real assistance.

Two hours into the flight, without any warning all the oxygen masks dropped down on the left side of the plane. I was sitting on the right. If there was a major problem with the pressurization system, those on the right side of the plane would have only a few seconds remaining. Was it simply a malfunction? I discounted a third possible explanation, that the whole thing was a joke, when I recalled that I had not since arriving in Russia observed anyone laughing about anything. Whatever the reason, the event caused considerable concern, with everyone trying to grab the nearest available mask. A bearded giant on my side of the plane reached over to the left side and completely wrenched the mask from its attachments. The hostesses, who had obviously become accustomed to such malfunctions calmly restored order – we were clearly not in need of oxygen.

I was now too exhausted to wonder about those who had pulled out what looked like bathmats and were kneeling in the aisle of the plane rocking in prayer. Was it gratitude, or just the time of the day? It might just have been a more comfortable alternative to the seating provided on this flight.

At this point I regretted not having put my hip flask (medicinal of course) in my jacket pocket. My hand luggage had slid under the seats behind and was irretrievable. I couldn't face the coffee or the bread offered either, but fortunately I had been warned about food on public transport in Russia and was armed with 36 Snickers bars, one of which was in my jacket.

The flight took only five and a half hours and I was wondering if I could stay on board during refuelling but by various means suddenly realized this *was* Irkutsk – we had not stopped to refuel at all. The last of the Canadians was disappearing out the exit, so I got off quickly and followed the crowd to what I thought was the domestic terminal. I failed to notice that the Canadians were not amongst those I was following. They were obviously familiar with the airport layout and had headed in the opposite direction, where international travellers were required to exit.

Having mistakenly followed all the people who face East, with their strange countenances, I found myself in an enormous airplane hanger, murky with cigarette smoke and full of people I could only regard as sinister, with their long beards and unusual facial characteristics. I was very ill at ease, but to my enormous relief was approached by a smiling, Western-dressed Dr Andrei Schapov.

He had been waiting at the International Arrivals lounge where I had failed to appear, so he was now very relieved to have found me. I think he was surprized at the pleasure with which I greeted him. Of course I didn't bother him with my problems, except to say that my luggage should be here somewhere but that I could not find a luggage carousel anywhere. He explained that this terminal was only for Russians with no checked baggage.

My suitcase had not come off the plane at Irkutsk, and it now seemed very unlikely it had come off at Moscow. So then began what could only be described as a farce entitled "Finding the Bag". Out of politeness I provided my hosts with hollow assurances that I was not in the least concerned about finding my baggage. "You have never lost your luggage in Russia", they replied.

Dr Schapov and the interpreter, Svetlana, guided me to a car which was to take us to the Sanatorium at Lake Baikal. Until recently the Sanatorium was the centre for the rehabilitation of the Russian wounded from the Afghanistan war. I did not know if Irkutsk was a typical remote Russian city, but during the two-hour ride to Lake Baikal I did not see anything that did not need repair. I thought of an Alaskan-style shanty town, with old wooden dwellings dating back 150 years. Here the buildings had obviously been ornate once, but were now unpainted and rarely vertical. The weight of snow on the roofs has caused all but the most sturdy to yaw to one side or the other. Communal water pumps were scattered along the road frontage and the roads – and most of the cars – were in an appalling state. The buildings in the commercial area were all dilapidated, with plaster falling from both interior and exteriors. No one person owned them so no one seemed to care or have pride in them.

While driving to Baikal Svetlana explained that the course I was to give had been advertised in Moscow, St Petersburg and several other cities. There was an ever-growing waiting list. The organizers were manual medicine practitioners and all the participants would be doctors.

On arriving at the Sanitorium I was taken to my lodge. This building had been constructed to house President Eisenhower for the Summit with Khrushchev in 1960 which had been cancelled when the American spy-plane with pilot Gary Powers was shot down over Russian territory. The building was sumptuously furnished and I had it to myself. I was provided with a housekeeper and a full-time interpreter in Svetlana. Things were looking up and at least I had my hand luggage. Two bottles of Vodka on my writing desk welcomed me.

My joy was short lived as my toilet did not work, and when I turned on the bath I had to bale out four or five gallons of rust before the water flowed. Nothing would go down the plughole. But at least I did now have someone with whom I could talk, and by my second day, feeling a little more rested and relaxed, I was able to take in the beauty of this desolate place. The house overlooked the frozen Lake Baikal. Snow covered and softened everything I could see outside. Irkutsk, with a population of 600,000, was 40 miles away.

My bath was a treat. It was seven feet by three feet and had the capacity to contain a young hippopotamus (as I lay in it I was reminded of the similarity). I had just emerged from my wallowing and was drinking a cup of instant coffee with long-life milk and saccharin, and a wholemeal biscuit, congratulating myself on having had the foresight to bring these delicacies with me, when a knock indicated I had not been forgotten.

Svetlana seemed slightly agitated. She asked if there was anything I required, but before I could answer she explained that there were problems with the Russian army in Moscow and that I should not be alarmed if the radio or television revealed gunfire, demonstrations and violence in that city. She said I was quite safe here as there were no such problems in Siberia. Their government did not agree with Moscow. Remembering from history lessons the plight of the Czar and his family in 1917 I asked Svetlana if this was another revolution. She assured me she would keep me informed of events, but in the meantime I was expected in the banquet room for dinner with the directors of the Rehabilitation Centre and the President of the Siberian branch of the Russian Academy of Medical Sciences, Dr Koleshnikov. Had he invented the automatic rifle of that name?

I apologized for having to wear the same clothing I had arrived in, albeit now clean, but Svetlana assured me everyone knew about my luggage plight. At least I had my toilet bag and razor and, most importantly, my slides.

After a very pleasant evening meal of cold meats and cheese accompanied by large quantities of vodka, I retired to my room and reflected on the evening's conversation. Inflation was increasing at the rate of seven per cent each month. The salaries of the medical and other staff were being so eroded that their 14,000 roubles per month equated to around US$50. Everyone was very concerned about the economy.

At lunch the following day we were to meet with a high Siberian Government official. He wished to present me with some sort of proposal, the detail of which I knew nought. On that occasion, though, he appeared for only two minutes, apologized, saying there has been a major upheaval in Moscow and he must attend an emergency meeting of some sort, and that he hoped to meet me privately at 5 p.m. the next day. I could only wait and wonder.

Lunch went on, without our host but with much vodka. From time to time Svetlana advised me of the general nature of the conversation. The assembled company, eight or ten all told, didn't seem to be very alarmed about the military situation, even though they said it was serious. They were used to crises and seemed to patiently await the outcome – seeking solace in the warmth of vodka. It made sense in this environment. The Russians grizzled about politics much as we do in New Zealand, but they appeared to be very happy on the whole. Unlike the company, I was not used to revolutionary dramas and I started wondering how I might be affected. Certainly my trip was badly timed and I felt rather stressed but at the same time excited by it all, but another vodka, and then another, helped. They were very friendly people and after the vodka they all laughed a lot, and seemed very pleased to have me with them. I had been put in palatial accommodation and was treated as a VIP in every way.

The following morning when I was being shown the lecture room, I noted that I was the object of intense curiosity. Many of the patients of the rehabilitation centre somehow appeared with perhaps their entire families and had lined up to see me as though I were some sort of celebrity. It turned out that they all had back problems and hoped they would be seen by me. They had apparently been told I was from New Zealand and that I had lost my luggage, and I was told that many were trying to joke with me – in Russian of course – about it.

The lecture hall seemed satisfactory but I immediately noticed that there was only one microphone – between myself, Svetlana and the patient. Without microphones the audience would not hear the patient and Svetlana would not be able to interpret. Anxiety grew in me as I was all too aware of the high expectations of all around me. And worse was to come. The projector was a long cartridge type and held only 50 slides. They only had two cartridges. I could only disguise my irritation and the course began. Translating my presentation was initially difficult for Svetlana, who was not familiar with the terms we commonly use. Dr Schapov was able to assist her most of the time but he too was limited. I discovered that if I was quick enough, I could reload the used cartridge for the projector during translation periods, but halfway through the morning the projector refused entirely to comply with the controls. An assistant had been advancing the slides at my signal but now he had to manually advance them using a screwdriver. By midday I was convinced that continuing with the projector was futile so I abandoned it altogether. After all, I was sure by now that few of the 60 doctors present understood my slides anyway!

After lunch came the patients. What disasters would I encounter? Did they have malingerers? Would the symptoms of a Russian with sciatica or referred pain centralize? Was I covered against malpractice? How would I deal with a sentence in the salt mines?

The first was a small man called Nicholai. His back pain had ceased months ago, at which time leg pain had started and was now severe. For demonstration purposes I had him sitting with his back to the audience and facing myself. He was sitting slouched, very slouched, and described severe leg pain in his buttock and calf. While he was still seated I drew his lumbar spine into an extended position, held it for a couple of minutes and asked about his pain. Svetlana translated that his leg pain had stopped, for the first time in five months, but he now felt midline back pain again. Oh how lucky I was. A posterior derangement no less, and reducible I concluded. True to the method following centralization of such symptoms, Nicolai was symptom free by the fifth day on a programme of extension and posture correction. On the final day he gave me a small present to show his gratitude I was sure he could ill afford to do so and was touched.

The second patient was Vladimir. He had had back and leg pain for three months and it was increasing. He was symptom free only when sitting and I observed that he sat bent forward. When he stood or walked or lay in bed the pain returned. Correcting his sitting posture produced an arc of severe pain in the back and leg as his lumbar spine moved from flexion to extension. On achieving and maintaining the erect posture he remained symptom free. On standing he also remained symptom free. I had him to return to the flexed sitting position for a few minutes and asked him to stand. His symptoms returned and standing was once more a continuously painful experience. I asked him to walk and all became clear. He walked leaning forwards. All it took for him to become symptom free was to correct the standing posture to exclude his forwards tilt. He would have to learn, or relearn that position to remain pain-free. *Quad erat demonstrandum.*

Russian patients were just like patients everywhere else it seemed. Spurred on with such early success, I treated eight patients on the first day. There were no failures. Over five days I saw 21 patients. Had I not seen so many, the group would never have had the opportunity to witness the nature of anterior derangement, nerve root adherence and entrapment and four spectacular reductions of derangement. Only one patient was unimproved, a triumph no less for didactic teaching and demonstration.

At the end of the first day I asked about my suitcase, but there was no news. At five I was to meet with the government official, Mr Pimanov. I was curious to learn about my special assignment. Pimanov, a deputy in the house of Delegates in the Central Government, had asked to see me privately. He apparently had a rather serious problem with his neck. He had most unusual symptoms, so unusual that I decided not to apply any external forces to his neck. No movements affected his pain, which was a warning that there could be a more serious problem. I suggested to him that X-rays would be a good idea; strangely he had not yet been X-rayed. He would arrange the pictures of his neck the following day and arranged to see me at the end of the week.

Some days later, this charming and vibrant man, took a party of us to dinner at a beautiful lodge set in the forest on the edge of Lake Baikal. Naturally there was much drinking of Vodka. In fact, as everyone present proposed a toast, many glasses had been downed. There was a ritual to this welcome. Firstly the senior officials from both the Government and the rehabilitation centre proposed a toast to me, then the Institute and then New Zealand. Then the respective wives followed. They raised glasses and toasted firstly Joy, then my father, my mother, then finally the new treatment method. Some seven or eight vodkas were downed and thus the evening continued with increasing merriment. Speeches ran into hearty singing of what I imagined were Russian folksongs.

As the course at the rehabilitation centre continued, the patients responded predictably and I began to feel very positive about my visit. The rapid reversal of the patients' disorders continued to amaze the group, and indeed me on one or two occasions. It reaffirmed my faith in the methods. Every patient was very anxious to get better, in contrast to some of our patients in New Zealand, and certainly in the USA where it was often more profitable to remain with pain.

I could not believe my luck. A patient with pain in the coccyx became symptom free merely as a result of being shown how to sit upright. A woman who had experienced pain for two years only at night, recovered almost completely following extension in lying. Patients seen over the previous days remained better. Marie, a lady of 70 Russian winters who could not stand erect, had had sciatica for two months. By the fifth day her pain was gone.

I saw the last of the patients and realized I had never seen as many centralize or reduce pain as rapidly or as completely as has occurred on this course. There had really only been one failure – a lady with coccydinia, the pain of which reappeared as miraculously as it disappeared.

On the last day of the course almost every patient brought me a gift, some very simple handmade presents – carvings or polished stone. Others were embarrassingly expensive.

My luggage actually appeared on the fifth day. I arrived back at my lodge after the course and there it was. I am not sure that anyone really noticed my limited wardrobe, but it was a huge relief to be able to change. It was bitterly cold and I now knew why the Russians, both men and women, wear their lovely fur hats, coats and boots. Men did not wear fine leather shoes; they would be ruined quickly in the winter snow and ice and as sealed footpaths were rare and there was often deep mud on the paths and roads. My own shoes were hopelessly inadequate for winter in Irkutsk.

On the fifth day I was interviewed for Siberian Radio and in the afternoon interviewed for Eastern Siberian television. My presence in Russia has been reported in Moscow and in Leningrad newspapers and people were calling up from all over the place seeking treatment, or husbands or wives calling seeking treatment for their spouses. The physical treatments most often provided in Russia had been the typical spa type, with hydrotherapy followed by massage. In recent years the European Manual Medicine group had introduced techniques of mobilization and manipulation. These courses became popular but the level of expertise attained was probably varied.

Many quaint methods of diagnosis were still used by Russian doctors. For instance, whilst trying to converse with one of the women physicians on the course, another doctor (male) pulled a copper divining rod from his pocket. After running the rod down her spine from occiput to coccyx he proceeded to advise her that she had had a gynaecological problem and headaches. She agreed that this was so but stated that most of her women patients had at some time had gynaecological problems and headaches, and then told him in Russian to get lost. At least that was the immediate effect of her terse communication.

My slide assistant in the course was also a accomplished pianist and every lunchtime he offered us a feast of Russian folk music. He was joined by a basso profundo of some 250 lbs in weight. The rhythm and liveliness of Russian folk music enticed all present to join in the performance. One very ancient character with a beard to his belt line produced a violin and away they all went in another round of music and singing. Everyone, it seemed, knew all the songs. In the corridors in the floors below, someone could be heard playing the piano-accordion and rattling out more folk tunes for an audience. They seemed to love this form of entertainment and relied very little on television.

It was time to leave this strange and wonderful place behind. Andre Shapov took me aside at our last meal together to tell me that Mr Pimanov was found to have cancer of the lungs and it had spread to his spine and other organs. I flew from Irkutsk the following day, having been made an honorary Doctor of the Siberian Branch of the Russian Academy of Medical Sciences and warmly invited to return.

The final of my many Russian dramas was when the taxi from Domodedovo to Sheremetyevo was stopped by soldiers. We were not allowed to enter the city, but I was delighted to hear that we must take the direct rather than the scenic route to the airport.

I had such mixed feelings about this experience, but I shall always remember with great warmth my visit to Russia.

Recently I heard that a plane had crashed leaving Irkutsk airport, killing all 186 passengers and crew. I could not help but wonder if it was the plane I had been on.

CHAPTER 12

THE ACCIDENT COMPENSATION SAGA

Over the years it had became very apparent to me that in New Zealand we had created a problem with back-pain patients. The conditions within then internationally highly regarded New Zealand health system seemed almost to perpetuate chronic back pain. Was our much-lauded no-fault accident compensation system in fact consigning many with chronic back pain to the scrap heap? With its generous levels of income support in a time of high unemployment, many were accepting and preferring their lot on accident compensation rather than the much lower payments provided by the dole! The Accident Compensation Corporation, ACC as it became known, was created in 1972 and provided insurance cover for injury by accident.

Viewing my clinical records around 1987 revealed to me that before 1973 two out of every three patients could not remember a reason for the onset of their problem, but that now two out of every three patients could distinctly recall a recent back injury. The word was out – if the patient could recall an "accident", almost any ache and pain would qualify them for free treatment, so many now attributed their back pain to an accident. This significant shift appeared to have created a problem that could only get worse. For clinicians this was an unexpected and unwelcome complication, although a few of the scallywags encouraged patients to "remember" some forgotten fall or lift. Our clinic had a fairly constant stream of patients who had been off work and on ACC for long periods. They were referred to me by their GPs. About two of every three of these ACC patients would respond and could go back to work. However, ACC's payment of weekly compensation instead of rehabilitation was not about to change because a few outpatients received benefit from a months' treatment at Kelvin Chambers.

In 1987 I had sought information from ACC statistics officers to confirm my suspicions. The statistics officer was not in the policymaking loop and she unwittingly let the cat out of the bag by stating that ACC had ceased funding for rehabilitation because of the number of long-term injured. The ACC, without advertising the fact, later closed three of four rehabilitation centres they had been supporting in New Zealand.

By 1989 there were over 14,000 workers with back problems in New Zealand who had been off work for more than two years, were being paid weekly compensation but were not being provided with any meaningful rehabilitation. Some of those were actually able to work but were abusing the system. Clinicians well trained in my methods could reliably identify those with treatable back pain and treat them with a high success rate. We could identify the non-genuine cases. The benefits to patients and a generous accident compensation system alike were obvious.

Research was beginning to show that although most who suffered back pain improved after 10 or 12 weeks even without treatment, a substantial number, over 50 per cent, still had disabling pain a year after injury. Without the diagnosis, treatment and education that formed the cornerstone of my treatment method these patients had no way of reducing their recurring problems.

I believed that what was required was a concerted effort by ACC case managers to have the chronic back pain population assessed and to select the suitable cases for treatment using my method. I decided I would develop a residential research and rehabilitation centre and provide a residential programme that would treat patients for 12 consecutive days. It could also serve as a centre for postgraduate education for clinicians wishing to complete the McKenzie Institute International Diploma programme as places were limited. The Institute had a waiting list of doctors and therapists wishing to obtain the higher qualification. My initial attempt to establish this centre in the monastery overlooking Oriental Bay in Wellington in 1989 proved difficult and to avoid further delays over appropriate accommodation, in 1990 I settled for what we called The Lodge at the Inlet, half an hour north of Wellington.

I set about recruiting appropriate staff. I needed at least three full-time and two part-time physiotherapists, two gym instructors, two technical assistants, a supervising physician and, if possible, someone to carry out research. With $100,000 worth of specialist equipment and good residential facilities the Institute could provide the longer-term treatment, education and research needed for an effective rehabilitation programme. I believed I should be directly involved in the rehabilitation programme, and thus returned to full-time practice for six hours a day, six days a week, curtailing my heavy international teaching commitments to do so.

I recruited Maynard Williams, a senior lecturer in statistics and psychology at the Auckland Technical Institute, who was willing to join the team and was interested in further back-related projects. One of his special briefs was to investigate the validity and effectiveness of the McKenzie system in returning chronic back-injured workers to work fitness. It would also be an asset to have someone keeping an eye on any data the ACC might produce. I already had serious concerns regarding the motives of those at the top of that organization.

To complete the specialist team I asked my old friend Dr David Wright to provide quality control. His task was to ensure that patients were medically fit for what was a strenuous rehabilitation programme. He was also responsible for completing accurate assessment of patients, and ensuring that if ACC eventually participated in rehabilitation they would be aware that they could not "fiddle the books". David's wife Jennifer, a nurse, also assisted in supervision of the exercise programme.

Joy was now free to assist with the supervision of patients in the gymnasium and pool and Jan also joined the team, to administer treatments on the four Repex machines, designed specifically for the more chronic lower-back disorders.

Within a few weeks of the programme being advertised in New Zealand and internationally the first intake, of mainly private residential customers, arrived, some coming from as far afield as the United States and Australia as well as from within New Zealand. The results were as expected. Of the ten patients in the first intake, eight were either significantly improved or pain free on leaving.

Two of the ten patients were under ACC, who when billed $2,000 for the treatment, paid without demur. My push for greater ACC involvement in rehabilitation made no progress until about a year later, when they cautiously began paying for the treatment of selected patients at the Institute. They seemed pleased with the results and I was soon asked to help with an ACC back-pain publicity campaign. I was beginning to think I had succeeded in securing ACC's involvement in rehabilitation, but, to my surprize, another section of the ACC, supported by Legal Counsel Gerard McGreevy, claimed that the Institute's treatment programme fell outside ACC's statutory responsibilities – it was only allowed to pay for "rehabilitation", not for "treatment". Funding ceased. I had to face the fact that I had enemies in the ACC.

I decided to go political, over the heads of ACC officials. The ACC had a clear responsibility for rehabilitation, a concept that to most health professionals was synonymous with treatment. In March 1991 I went to see the Minister in charge of the ACC, the redoubtable Bill Birch. Mr Birch was known to be intent on reforming that body. Birch agreed to meet me and our CEO Lawrence Dott. Incredibly, ACC had not thought it necessary to advise the Minister that there were some 13,500 patients with back pain on its books who had not worked for more than two years. The Minister became interested and appeared sympathetic to our cause. ACC Chief Executive Jeff Chapman and his legal counsel McGreevy were also present at this meeting and I could see they were uncomfortable. But my case was simple: why was the ACC not supporting an Institute that could help reduce the Corporation's enormous earnings-related compensation payout of over NZ$250 million per annum, by identifying malingerers and restoring most patients to work-fit status – thus taking up to two-thirds of the chronic patients off the books?

I invited the Minister to visit the Lodge to see what we were doing and at the same time launch the new Repex equipment we had installed. A study in Canada had recently been published and showed that continuous movement of knee joints had caused cartilage lining of joints to repair, even after significant injury. With the help of Howard Wright in New Plymouth we designed the world's first Continuous Passive Movement equipment for the treatment of the lower back. We called this machine Repex (Repeated End-Range Passive Exercise). This equipment allowed the patient to completely relax while the machine moved them repeatedly into extension.

The Minister promised to re-establish the ACC's responsibility for rehabilitation and asked Chapman to move on with the programme and study. I'm sure there was opposition from behind the scenes, but the ACC set up a process that would ensure we were given a fair trial. Or so we thought at the time.

The ACC then called for a pilot project. They would compare four new rehabilitation programmes available. It was the breakthrough I had been hoping for. At our first meeting, however, the ACC's rehabilitation adviser, Lauretta Alessi, made the extraordinary statement that they had no intention of rehabilitating back patients if there was no work for them to go to. (This was a time of high unemployment in New Zealand.) I could not believe what I was hearing. This response from the person ostensibly directing rehabilitation of the injured raised serious doubts about the philosophy and aims of the Corporation. This was not the last time I was to hear ACC officials repeat that and make other statements that addressed neither the needs of patients nor the interests of taxpayers.

With the trial set up, I wrote to all the GPs and medical centres in New Zealand notifying them of the establishment of the rehabilitation unit and informing them that ACC would fund patients. They responded immediately. There were few of them who did not have patients who had been cast aside by the ACC and they were delighted to now have something to offer them. We received an immediate avalanche of requests – 180 in the first month – from all over the country.

In February 1992 the Minister's initiative allowed us to begin a pilot project for 200 patients for the ACC. We were allowed to recruit our own patients, to be subsequently approved by ACC.

In the first four months the Institute dealt with over 70 patients and, as predicted, we were able to restore more than 60 per cent of them to a work-fit state as measured by the ACC's own medical assessors. However, some officials were still obviously hostile, and on 30 September 1992 the ACC insisted the chronic back pain contract had to be rewritten or terminated. I was not impressed by this ultimatum when we were operating under a ministerial directive. I was willing to negotiate, but not under duress. To ensure that the programme ran smoothly I had personally attended the Centre for the whole of the period and pitched in whenever necessary. I had given my time and knowledge freely, and received no salary or other remuneration other than a free lunch daily at the Lodge.

It was all very soul-destroying but we had invested a great deal of energy in the centre and were prepared to do battle. I went to Russia for ten days amid all this confusion, but returned at the end of March 1993 ever more motivated to change the New Zealand situation.

Now we had to work our way through this new ACC crisis. I asked the Hon. Bill Jeffries, with his vast political experience, to act as my attorney. The Corporation then backed down, and we negotiated an acceptable new contract for the Centre's residential back study. With referrals coming from throughout New Zealand, the study confirmed that over 63 per cent of chronic back pain clients were rehabilitated to be capable of working and all patients were assessed by the ACC's own medical assessors. The Centre was able to demonstrate twice the recovery of function and mobility through its programme than any of the other three programmes being trialled.

GPs and specialists alike were delighted. Such was the level of referrals that the ACC by mistake or incompetence approved over 150 more patients than the study required and then, despite the positive results, accused the Institute of deliberately overrunning the agreed figure.

The hostility continued. The ACC now issued notice to us advising that as the Institute had failed to return those in the programme to full employment, it had failed to reach the target success rate. Contradicting this, in September 1993 the ACC had published information in medical publications about the success of their joint back study with the McKenzie Institute. The Corporation's research manager, Alan Woodside, went on to offer congratulations on the success of the venture, suggesting that the Corporation now "get on with business of rehabilitating all the back injured workers", and confirming plans for a second research contract.

This evidence of intent was important in allowing me to keep my team together. The ACC's new chief executive, Gavin Robbins, had, on the instructions of Minister Bill Birch, visited the Centre in November 1993. He brought with him several Board members and his legal counsel Gerard McGreevy, now the general manager in charge of research. Robbins' reaction seemed to assure the continuation of the programmes.

In December 1993 an ACC letter indicated planning for more research was under way. Jo Adams in the ACC back study management team confirmed that the Corporation had approved a new study, and in January indicated that a first intake of patients could be expected before the end of February 1994. Lawrence Dott and I decided on this basis to keep on the staff hired for the initial research. However, the ACC's draft contract revealed a major shift in their approach. The Corporation's clerical staff would now take over the identifying and recruiting of patients. This seemed odd. How could clerical staff determine the need or otherwise for rehabilitation? Nevertheless the ACC appeared committed to supporting a second study and sought the Institute's commitment to handling a minimum of 40 cases a month.

Committing to 40 patients a month had cost implications. The clinic had initially taken in private patients and was doing well, but in order to process 40 ACC patients a month it would have to cease taking private patients. The corporation now offered start-up on 15 April 1994 – the promised February start-up had not occurred.

The costs of retaining the staff, without remuneration from private patients or ACC put the Institute under financial stress, but knowing that 40 patients per month would be forthcoming we duly signed the contract for the second project.

As a charitable trust we could not borrow to cover expenses; the Institute had to depend on operational income, which the new contract appeared to provide. No patients appeared in April. None came in May. Finally in June, ACC referred six patients, another four in July and no prospects were planned for August. Later Gerard McGreevy was to claim credit for a special clause written into the contract, which we now became painfully aware of, that exempted the Corporation from liability for any failure to provide the 40 patients that the Institute had contracted to handle each month. We were in serious trouble; it would take time to publicize our reopening for private patients and we simply could not keep the staff on. With great sadness we had to close the Lodge.

In 1995 the Institute took the ACC to court, claiming compensation for its losses amounting to almost $300,000. The Corporation claimed that it did not have sufficient patients to supply the Institute and in any case it was not obliged to supply any at all. The Institute claimed that ACC officials had repeatedly assured them verbally that a second study would go ahead – "You must keep the Lodge open ready for a start in the New Year." We later learned that "a top official" in ACC ordered the destruction of documents relating to the ACC and the Institute just before the case was to be heard.

When Gerard McGreevy, Alan Woodside and Jo Adams took the stand for cross-examination and were reminded of their assurances and undertakings to myself and Lawrence, not surprisingly all three had a serious loss of memory, stating, on oath, that they could not recall.

The case, heard before a judge sitting alone, was decided in favour of the Institute. Justice McGechen found that the ACC had misled the Institute into assuming it could expect a continuing flow of patients. However, in his final judgment he was unable to determine our loss. We were stunned by this as our accountants had provided evidence of the financial losses sustained. Justice McGechan awarded the McKenzie Institute damages in the amount of $100. We appealed the decision but this was rejected by the Court.

Subsequently Prof David McLauchlan of the Law Faculty at Victoria University wrote an article in the *New Zealand Business Law Quarterly*, May 1998, that was highly critical of the reasoning of Justice McGechan and the three Appeal Court judges (Sir Ivor Richardson, and Justices Tipping and Keith), suggesting that the case was wrongly decided.

Three years after the closure of the Lodge rehabilitation programme the CEO of the ACC, Jeff Chapman, was jailed for fraud. Thirteen years later, McGreevy was persuaded to resign. Many who could have been helped had been greatly disadvantaged by his decision that they were not covered by the ACC for some reason or another. Many later received compensation after review of the process failures under his counsel.

Jeff Chapman, Gerard McGreevy and Loretta Alessi were responsible for this unfortunate policy which left thousands of people with back problems without treatment that could so easily have been provided and paid for by a fraction of the income-based compensation that ACC was paying out.

CHAPTER 13

THE McKENZIE INSTITUTE INTERNATIONAL

The news of the development and adoption of the McKenzie Method in North America spread rapidly. European physiotherapists attended US courses and took the news home to their various countries. Some of the founders of the Institute in the US contributed significantly to the development of branches worldwide. The first teaching faculty appointed in the United States – Kathy Hoyt, Dan Kelley, Greg Silva, Hugh Murray, Barbara Stone, Wayne Rath and Angelo di Maggio – were joined later by Mark Miller, Scott Herbowy, Robert Medcalf, Dana Greene, Elaine Gillman and Ron Bybee. Most of them were to spend many years developing the Institute. Wayne Rath and Angelo di Maggio eventually decided to go it alone.

While in Dallas in 1980 Dr Mooney introduced me to his secretary Ann Carlton who, as was her habit, took me under her wing and ensured my accommodation and meals were satisfactory. She was originally a physical therapist but had become Dr Mooney's office assistant and organized and ran projects for the orthopaedic department. I soon learned that Anne was an indispensable part of the Mooney family and had been assisting Vert for many years. She acquainted me with the various difficulties I would have to overcome in gaining recognition for a system so diametrically opposite to current thinking. Anne helped me enormously in my early years travelling in the United States and she has been the very competent behind-the-scenes organizer of most of the Institute Conferences, until retiring recently.

In the early 1980s, in addition to my own continuing North

American tours, I found the interest from European countries to be following the same pattern as occurred in the United States between 1977 and 1979. The word of the new method spread rapidly from Holland to Belgium, Germany, Denmark and Sweden. Clinicians found that MDT was so superior to the traditional methods in use currently and it was difficult for me to cope for the requests for education. Following my first visit to the United Kingdom in 1981 a branch of the Institute was formed only three years later by Malcolm Robinson, Peter Legeard and a New Zealander Juliette Moss who was living in England at that time. Later, Andrew Holdom, Jenny Ross and Fiona Farmer joined the teaching faculty. In 2000 a new CEO, Bridgette Crundwell, was appointed to take charge of the UK branch.

Stephen May, also based in the UK and who I have been working with since the mid 1980s, has an extraordinary knowledge of the scientific literature relating to musculo-skeletal disorders in general and the spine in particular and is an indispensable part of our organization. Stephen successfully completed his doctorate in 2008.

A branch in Canada followed in 1985, where my old friend Colin Davies was joined by Rikki Yamada and Phil Burchell. Later these three were joined by Sheila McBride, Daniele Poulin, Richard Rosedale and one of our star researchers Audrey Long. The Australian Institute was also established in 1985, by Helen Clare, Bev Dalziell and Gwynne Thomas. In 1986 a branch was formed in New Zealand, with Mark Laslett, Paula van Wijmen, Ace Neame, Tom Burgi Rob Reid and myself the founding members. Also in 1986, Jeanette Bissig and Reto Genuchi commenced teaching and formed a branch of the Institute in Switzerland. Almost every year since then a new branch has been formed as the method has spread internationally.

After my first visit to the United States, and in the early days of the US McKenzie Institute, the volume of mail had increased at a rate that justified the employment of a full-time secretary at home base in New Zealand, a luxury that I had never before considered. Unfortunately, the first person I engaged could not spell; my taped dictation was transformed into something between Esperanto and Pidgin English. For the month that she lasted I fell further and further behind. I then sought assistance from a secretarial service in Waikanae, and this served my needs for the next year or two. However, as time passed and the correspondence became even more voluminous, this also became inadequate.

Early in 1984 I had advertised a secretarial position in the local newspapers and Mrs Joanne Moffat arrived at End Farm for an interview. She had a very impressive CV and listed amongst her previous employers was the NZ Federation of Labour, a sole-charge position where she acted as secretary to the Secretary of the Federation; the NZ Airways Corporation (now known as Air New Zealand), where she acted as secretary to both the Chief Engineer and the Public Relations Manager; the NZ Police Department where she had the position of Supervisor of the typing pool; and a couple of part-time positions, one with the NZ Department of Education and another in the office of a senior Member of Parliament, both positions requiring fast typing skills.

Joanne was from Scotland. From our first meeting I knew that she would be eminently suitable for the job – to keep me up to date with the ever-increasing flow of invitations, record my future commitments, sort both the domestic and business accounts, and type out drafts of my writings. Joanne completed everything in the most meticulous fashion and was highly professional. Because telephone charges for international calls were very high at the time, we were still organising courses through the mail system and arrangements could take many weeks and much care and patience to complete.

It became increasingly clear to me that although reluctant to be seen to conform to the fad that was taking over the world, I had to consider the purchase of a computer and word processor. I thought at that time they were entirely separate machines. While I found such a radical step to have some merit, I was unenthusiastic about the adoption of email, now being touted as the electronic communication system for the future. So a computer was purchased and both Joanne and I set about learning the intricacies of word-processing. Learning computer terminology and the difference between hard copy, soft copy, hard drive and software was part of the challenge. We quickly came to recognize the potential value of this wonderful tool. Email, however, was out of the question and could wait indefinitely, or so I thought, but the necessity for the speedy communication it offered won out, and a year or so later we succumbed. Our progress was, of course, transformed by the efficiency of this technology.

My daughter Jan and her husband's management of Spinal Publications from their home was a huge weight off my mind and allowed me to focus on the many jobs I was involved in, including my trips to the United States and Europe demonstrating for several months at a time, as well as managing and organising the Institute. It was nevertheless growing quite beyond me. Limited space at the office at End Farm was also limiting our efficiency; Joanne's files stretched from wall to wall and from floor to ceiling.

Later in Joanne's first year we acquired office and warehouse space in Parata Street, Waikanae, which was also ideal for the manufacture, assembly, and marketing and distribution of the low-back and neck supports which I needed for my own patients but which were at that time unobtainable commercially. The extra space also provided accommodation for the offices of Spinal Publications and allowed for the storage for Spinal's stock. A further and probably the most important benefit derived from the purchase of the Parata Street premises was that the building allowed for the expansion of the McKenzie Institute International offices.

In 1988, on 10 June, with assistance from Sir Jack Marshall the New Zealand Back Foundation, a charitable trust, was created. Sir Jack was the trust's first chairman. The function of the Foundation was to market the spinal supports to provide funds for treatment of patients, the education of clinicians and research into spinal mechanical disorders. Under the name of Backcare, hundreds of thousands of dollars were raised for these purposes. Following the death of Sir Jack, Sir David Beattie, a former Governor General of New Zealand, took over the patronage of the Back Foundation. He was followed by orthopaedic surgeon Peter Hunter and the Foundation continued to provide research funding until 2005.

In 1989 an old friend, Patrick Thomas, expressed interest in my proposal that he manage Spinal Publications and take on the role of CEO of the Institute. Jan had decided to take on the role of receptionist at our newly established clinic at the Ropata Medical Centre in Lower Hutt. Two years later, when Patrick had just become familiar with the complexities of the book marketing trade and the Institute, he died in tragic circumstances. Again I took the helm at the Institute, which was rapidly becoming more than a full-time job. The search began for a replacement for Patrick. That person would have to be taught the complexities that allowed the commercial aspects of book promotion to be kept at arm's length and independent from the scientific and professional activities of myself and the Institute, not an easy task.

Lawrence Dott was also an acquaintance of old. We had not met often prior to a chance meeting in 1991 when I learned that he had recently changed jobs and was not entirely settled in his new position. Lawrence was very presentable, well educated in the business world and was definitely going to be a top contender. He said he would think about my offer.

A few days later, on 1 March 1991, Lawrence Dott became CEO of the McKenzie Institute International – a position he holds to this day. Relieved from the responsibility of managing the daily affairs of the Institute, I felt that a tremendous burden had been lifted from my shoulders. He gradually became familiar with the affairs of the Institute and took on the diplomatic negotiation of our complex international relationships. The success of the McKenzie Institute International can largely be attributed to Lawrence's steady hand at the helm.

Now began a significant reorganization of the Institute's structure and management. The various branches were provided with a manual of policies and procedures to be followed in accordance with their contracts with the Institute. A Director of Education was appointed to ensure the integrity of the teaching and the true method that had been perfected. Some teachers had introduced changes or variations to what was supposed to be presented to paying students, and we had had several angry clinicians complaining that they had attended our programme to learn precisely what Robin McKenzie had discovered and how he practised and not the personal ideas of their tutor.

The original courses I presented were confined to demonstrating the method on lower back problems. This was eventually expanded and became two separate programmes to teach the procedures of diagnosis and treatment of the neck and middle spine. Later, as the demand continued to increase for more education and hands-on learning, a third course was added which included laboratory practice. A fourth course added problem solving and further hands-on practice. Following the publication of the text covering the application of the McKenzie Method to the human extremities the demand for education resulted in the development of a fifth course. All of the course materials have now been standardized for each branch across the world.

Paula van Wijmen, who had begun the process of structuring our lectures and demonstrations soon after the Institute was formed in 1983, was followed by Rodney Grant. In 1990 it was decided that a formal Institute Diploma programme would be commenced to provide the right level of theoretical and practical education.

The purpose was to train individuals from participating centres to a level that would enable them to return to their native environment and teach their compatriots the correct use of MDT in their own language. Rodney was to lead the first diploma course in New Zealand, which was sited at the Rehabilitation Centre at the Lodge at the Inlet. Among those attending during that period were Ron Bybee, Dana Greene, Mark Miller, Scot Herbowy, Gary Jacob, Robert Medcalf, Nico de Bruine from the Netherlands, Dan Zu Zang from China, Osola Ayanniyi from Nigeria and Vinod Agrawal from India. We were becoming a truly international organization.

Rodney Grant was followed by David Poulter who was followed by Helen Clare, and in 1999 she became the Institute's first Director of Education. Helen was a New Zealander living at the time in Sydney. She achieved what I could only have dreamed of in our education process – perfection! We now have a joint venture in distance learning with Otago University, where Stuart Horton is our instructor, and in 2010 will commence a similar programme with Dundee University, where Jenny Ross and John Thompson will be joint lecturers. In addition, we provide clinical education at various centres in New Zealand, Denmark and the United Kingdom. Scott Herbowy and Mark Miller established a Diploma facility in Austin, Texas, which has produced many fine graduates. More recently, Todd Edelson set up another Diploma facility in New Jersey. Worldwide, all 28 branches and associated faculty of the McKenzie Institute International provide identical educational programmes and diagnostic and therapeutic demonstrations. Helen completed her doctorate in early 2008 and has been involved in several studies on the value of MDT. She was, and remains, an outstanding asset to the Institute.

Juergen Schmid had first invited me to Germany in 1983. He recruited Jan Kuiper and a branch was formed in 1993 when Tom Burgi, fluent in German, joined the group. Ron Donelson, the orthopaedic surgeon mentioned earlier, made significant progress in European medical and surgical communities in promoting the value of MDT. He presented three courses to doctors in Denmark, three in Italy, four in the Netherlands, and one each in Estonia and Finland. The resultant surge in the spread of knowledge of MDT in these countries has also seen an increase in the publication of studies relevant to the system. His many scientific papers published in peer-reviewed journals demonstrated the reliability and predictive value of centralizing pain. His book about my method, *Rapidly Reversible Low Back Pain*, exposes the biases and prejudices that exist amongst some of the leading figures in back-pain research.

There were many in Europe who made lasting contributions to the Institute's growth and wellbeing. In Holland, two outstanding figures in physiotherapy were Bert van Kuick and Nico de Bruine. They organized my first courses and have since the formation of the Benelux branch in

1991 led the Institute in Holland, Belgium and Luxemburg. They were joined by Hans van Helvoit who commenced teaching in 1993.

All three hold senior lecturer status in the Institute Bert also serves on the Institute's Advisory Council. Other staunch supporters were found in Sweden where Margarita Myrenberg and Lars Dagerfield were most prominent. Thanks to the contributions of Uffe Lindstrom, Ole Meyer, Lena Skytte, Charlotte Krog and Sten Olsen in Denmark the Danish guidelines for diagnosis and treatment of low back pain were the first to give the various aspects of MDT official recognition by the Danish Ministry of Health.

Sara Leutchford, Antoine Gemayel, Sandro Aina and Antonio Lenzini of Italy began the process of educating their countrymen and women even before the Italian branch was established in 1991.

In 1993 branches of the McKenzie Institute International were formed in Nigeria, where Olusola Ayanniyi is our representative, and in Finland, where Tuija Siitonen and Sinikka Kilpikoski have developed strong research-based branches. The Institute branch in Greece was founded in 1995 by Georgos Spanos who to this day still calls me "father". His partner Katerina Damanaki acts as the branch manager. Brazil followed in 1996; Jose Liberato and his wife Yara have created such interest in the McKenzie Method that Rio hosted the Institute biennial international conference in 2009.

Thomas Stengart a senior specialist physician in Poland developed a strong branch and interest in MDT following my visit there in 1994. The Polish Government has recently announced that it will fund the training of 300 clinicians in MDT.

France followed in 1998 when Gabor Sagi developed widespread interest in MDT. France was one of the few countries where I did not present courses and initiate the interest myself. In Hungary, Scott Herbowy from our US faculty, who was fluent in Hungarian, was instrumental in the introduction of the method to that country. In 1995, Stacey Lyon was appointed CEO of the United States branch of the Institute and has created, and continues to develop, a strong and ever-growing organization. In 1999 we added Saudi Arabia to the list, with Jabr Al-Jabr leading the way.

The Institute was formed in 1982 in the United States of America by doctors and physiotherapists involved in the teaching of the McKenzie Method of Mechanical Diagnosis and Therapy.

The formation of the McKenzie Institute arose from the need to ensure that the highest standards of teaching were provided to those wishing to learn the McKenzie Method. Following inauguration, the Institute established its international headquarters in New Zealand during 1984. The branches and year of formation follow:

1982	USA	1995	Hellas / Cyprus
1984	United Kingdom	1996	Brazil
1985	Canada		Poland
	Australia	1998	France
1986	New Zealand	1999	Saudi Arabia
	Switzerland	2000	Croatia
1990	The Netherlands	2002	Japan
1991	Italy	2003	Czech Republic
	Belgium	2004	Norway
	Luxembourg	2008	Argentina
1992	Sweden		Slovenia
1993	Germany		
	Denmark		
	Nigeria		
	Russia		
	Finland		
	Hungary		

Discussions with Head Office are currently underway for the formation of Branches in China, Egypt, India, Israel, Lebanon, South Africa and Spain.

In 2008 a separate International Branch of the Institute was established specifically for MDT Education to Doctors of Chiropractic and Doctors of Osteopathy. This branch is managed by the Institute's Head Office.

In addition to those countries where branches have been or are being established, McKenzie MDT Education is also currently provided in Qatar, United Arab Emirates, Mexico, Hong Kong and Bangladesh.

Early in my career I realized that research into the theories and methods would be essential if recognition was to be achieved at some time in the future. Thankfully, many of the faculty members of the Institute have taken up the challenge and in the intervening period hundreds of studies of MDT have emerged in the scientific literature on back problems. That momentum was given significant impetus in 2007, when under the guidance of Dr Ted Dreisinger, a Vietnam War veteran, the International Mechanical Diagnosis and Therapy Research Foundation became a reality and is now accumulating funds from donations to sponsor independent research. Ted has been a pillar of strength to me from the time we first met at the American Back Society meeting – The Quiet Revolution – in Boston in 1992. Ted has spoken at many of our conferences and his guidance over the years has been indispensable.

Many members of the McKenzie Institute have responded to the need for research and literature to validate and explain principles of MDT. Early contributors who laid a solid foundation include Ron Donelson, Vert Mooney and Radislav Stankovic. Elegantly designed and presented studies were added by Mark Werneke and Audrey Long. Others who have contributed over the years include Greg Silva, Paula Van Wijman, Mark Laslett, Robert Medcalf, Helen Razmjou, Rikki Yamada, Bruce Haugar, Ron Bybee, Carol Dionne, Sinikka Kilpikoski, Stephen May, Helen Clare, Lene Skytte, Lars Dagerfeldt, Cheryl Hefford, Sharon Young, Richard Rosedale, Mark Rosenfeld and Alessandro Aina. A comprehensive list of references supporting MDT is available on the McKenzie Institute International website www.mckenziemdt.org.

In 1999 I received an invitation to introduce MDT to Japan. The course was to commence in late March 2000 and I asked Robert Medcalf, from the senior teaching faculty in the United States, to accompany me to the introductory course to be held at the Saitama Medical Hospital University near Tokyo in Japan. Physiotherapist Yoshi Iwasada prepared and organized the venue and patients. Although Robert and I were well accustomed to seeing the changes that we could make, this was a completely new experience for the Japanese therapists. They were very excited about this new system of diagnosis and treatment. On that visit Robert and I were entertained royally by the Japanese and, apart from letting our hair down at a Karaoke club, we were generally well-behaved in Japan.

Since that course Yoshi has obtained the Institute Diploma and has become a pillar of strength for MDT in Japan. Yoshi, with orthopaedic surgeon Toshiro Ishibashi MD acting as chairman, formalized a Japanese branch of the Institute in 2002. Another Japanese orthopaedic surgeon, Koki Anabuki, has now written a textbook in Japanese describing in detail the McKenzie MDT method.

In 2000 I received an invitation from the Chinese Ministry of Health to teach at the Beijing Hospital and start the process of educating physicians involved in rehabilitation in that vast country. I decided to take with me one of our senior teaching faculty, Dana Greene from the US. At the airport in Beijing I was met by Cynthia Gu, a physician attached to the Rehabilitation section of the hospital. Cynthia spoke English well and interpreted for all the patients and at the lectures. She has subsequently led the education process in China and assisted in the political manoeuvring so necessary to achieve the formal development of the branch.

The Chinese experience was amazing. Beijing Hospital is where senior Chinese Government officials seek treatment, Chairman Mao having been one the most notable patients. Nothing resembling my system of management for back pain had ever been seen there before. The course of demonstration began 9 October 2000 and was extended to five days to allow for the extra interpretation time needed.

As usual Dana and I demonstrated with some of the problem patients at the hospital. One of them, a cardiac specialist, was suffering from severe sciatica. His X-rays showed an extremely large disc protrusion and he was scheduled to have surgery a week later. With his pain centralized on the first session, he was a classic candidate for the McKenzie Method. He lost his leg pain in 24 hours and was almost totally free of pain by the fifth day. The 44 doctors in the demonstration room had seen the extent of the disc protrusion and could not believe the patient would recover without surgery; they considered the cardiologist to be wasting his time with these new exercises.

Dana and I had a wonderful time and were treated very well. Apart from our failure to realize that in China 6.30 for dinner *means* 6.30 for dinner, we were otherwise well behaved. Over a sumptuous dinner, the President of the Beijing Hospital asked me if I would return and teach all the Rehabilitation doctors in China this new method. I asked how many this would involve, and swallowed several times when he responded with the figure of several hundred thousand. I told him we would be agreeable to this proposal and would enter into an agreement, indicating though, that this education process might take some time! Educational seminars are due to commence in China in 2009.

In 1989, in Newport Beach California, the McKenzie Institute International held its first conference. Clinicians were invited from various countries where my system was well developed. Several world-renowned back-pain authorities were invited to attend as guest speakers. Among them was Richard Deyo, who is the author of many studies on back pain. Deyo spoke again at the Institute's conference in Queenstown, New Zealand in 2007. One of our own most strident critics, Alf Nachemson, gave his first presentation at the Institute's conference in Ottawa in 2001. As time passed Nachemson slowly warmed to our method and eventually announced, to our delight, that we were on the right track. The first meeting was so successful we decided we would hold them on a regular basis, and it gave me great satisfaction to find we could attract large numbers to these events. Since then international conferences have been held every two years – in Dallas, Toronto, Cambridge, Philadelphia, Maastricht, Ottawa, Rome, Crete, Queenstown and, in 2009, Rio de Janeiro. At each one we have had the best speakers the planet has to offer. Dr Mooney, who was chairman at many of our conferences, has spoken at them all. He has also served on the Board of Trustees of the McKenzie Institute International since 1986.

The conferences have also offered the opportunity for the faithful followers to gather from around the world. So not only has it been a time for serious scientific discussion of things mechanical relating to the spine and extremities, but it has also included faculty meetings for those teaching courses around the world. The size of these meetings has grown from the early handful to well over a hundred faculty. The conferences have also provided some very enjoyable social events. One with special meaning was the dinner party in New Zealand in 2007 when we celebrated the 25th anniversary of the founding of the Institute. Over 100 attended and all were in the costumes of their home countries.

It has become a tradition for the Institute to present an award during the conferences. The award has been known as the Extension Award and it has been given to individuals who have made significant contributions to furthering MDT. The award is a bronze lady lying on her stomach doing press-ups. These are the recipients to date.

Extension Award recipients

1990	Vert Mooney, MD	United States
1991	Ron Donelson, MD	United States
1992	Dan Kelley, PT, Dip. MDT	United States
1993	Paula Van Wijmen, PT, Dip. MDT	New Zealand
1994	Mark Laslett, PT, Dip. MDT	New Zealand
1995	Radislav Stankovic, RPT	Sweden
1996	David Poulter, PT, Dip. MDT	United States
1997	Ronald Donelson, MD	
	Charles Aprill, MD	
	Robert Medcalf, PT, Dip. MDT	
	William Grant, EdD	United States
1998	Kathleen M. Hoyt, PT, Dip. MDT	United States
1999	Audrey Long, PT, Dip. MDT	Canada
2000	Mark Werneke, PT, Dip. MDT	United States
2001	Stover Snook, MD	United States
	Helen Razmjou, PT, Dip. MDT	Canada
2002	Stephen May, PT, Dip. MDT	United Kingdom
	Helen Clare, PT, Dip. MDT	Australia
	John Sullivan, PhD	New Zealand
2003	Kristian Larsen, PT	Denmark
	Tom Petersen, PT	Sweden
	Sinikka Kilpikoski, MSc, PT, Dip. MDT	Finland

2004	Audrey Long, PT, Dip. MDT	Canada
2005	Ted Dreisinger, PhD, FACSM	United States
2006	Helen Clare, PhD (USyd), PT, Dip. MDT	Australia

Under Lawrence Dott's management from New Zealand the Institute was transformed, leaving me, in the later 90s and into the new century, free to concentrate on breaking new ground in countries such as China and Japan. I could relax knowing that the organization was in good shape and hands. We have never had to canvass our wares; clinicians came to us pleading for help after reading or hearing of the method and its effectiveness. Applications for our education programmes came in from all corners of the world in a never-ending stream. Many of these requests were from countries such as Nigeria, Bangladesh, Croatia and Bosnia. Although they could not afford to pay the airfares or hotels for our instructors, we were determined to assist them and we used surplus monies derived from courses held in the United States and parts of Europe where course attendances were much higher.

I considered approaching the New Zealand Government for financial assistance to introduce the method in third-world countries, but we determined that the Institute could just break even without such support and we would avoid additional bureaucratic complications. The Accident Compensation Corporation debacle had taught us a bitter lesson.

The year 2003 saw the development of a branch in the Czech Republic, founded by Eva Novacova. Norway joined in 2004, followed by Argentina and Slovenia in 2008.

With this commitment to the cause by such strong and dedicated individuals and branches I had no trouble demonstrating the effectiveness of the McKenzie Method to clinicians all over the world.

This rapid growth, after all the years of frustration and seeming insurmountable opposition, was hard to believe. I could now see that clinicians were using mechanical diagnosis to deliver appropriate treatment to their patients all over the world. It became clear that MDT, against the odds, was going to survive; that my Mr Smith and I had brought about a very significant change in the way bad backs would be diagnosed and treated. It was widely regarded as a really important breakthrough in this field of medicine and now it would go on. How sweet it all was.

Despite my longstanding opposition to chiropractors and their widely held belief that all patients with spinal pain required manipulation and that spinal manipulation or adjustment could cure all manner of diseases in both adults and children, my attitude was significantly modified after a chiropractor by the name of Gary Jacob contacted me in 1990 to say that he was very impressed with what he had read in my first book. He was based in Los Angeles and had been using my system for several years with excellent results and he also found the philosophy behind the method to be compelling. Gary came to New Zealand in 1991 to sit the Institute Diploma Examination. Needless to say, he passed with flying colors.

This was a different kind of chiropractor to those I had met in the past. I was also fascinated by the words he chose and the manner in which he spoke. It sometimes took me until the next day to work out what he was actually saying, or I was just never able to work it out. Occasionally he would note my confusion and try to explain himself in simpler terms. As time passed I gradually came to comprehend what could almost be described as his lectures to me.

Gary wanted me to come to the United States and give demonstrations to his chiropractic colleagues. I knew that my reputation and earlier hostility to the chiropractic profession would precede me and was somewhat diffident about accepting this invitation. Gary assured me that there would be no hostility but I might face a degree of scepticism, which he believed would dissipate once the results showed through.

In February 1992 I accepted Gary's invitation to Los Angeles and appeared before a group of about 25 chiropractors who had been persuaded by Gary to front up to my course. I insisted that we have real patients for the course, because even the most sceptical of professionals were usually won over on witnessing the effect of the various manoeuvres. The patients, as expected, demonstrated most of the characteristics I relied on to get the message across and the first education programme for chiropractors in the United States was a success. Since that time Doctors Gary Jacob and Stephen Heffner have continued with the slow process of convincing sceptical colleagues of the value of MDT and, amazingly, there are now many chiropractors in the United States practising the McKenzie Method.

In 2007 the McKenzie Institute International signed a joint-venture agreement with the National University of Health Sciences in Chicago. Courses in MDT will be taught by both Jacob and Heffner. The first presentations commenced in 2008 and will expand to include Chicago, Florida, Toronto and Harvard in 2009.

I could never have predicted this development would occur in my lifetime. I had gradually become more tolerant and inclusive of the chiropractic profession and they had shown a willingness to embrace a treatment method that they had long scorned as it was so different to their manipulation techniques. I believe, though, that the chiropractic profession's acceptance of MDT can only be to the benefit of all patients in their care.

Many physiotherapists both in New Zealand and abroad have voiced their concerns that teaching chiropractors will increase the competition for patients. It may well increase the competition, but the patient will be the better off for it and that, as far as I am concerned, is the only thing that matters.

So, after a century of antagonism and hostility, I feel enormous satisfaction in having built a bridge between these two groups. One day there will be only one profession with the responsibility for dispensing non-surgical care for spinal disorders. Will they be called chirotherapists or physiopractors? Who knows?

EPILOGUE

There has been both great pleasure and some heartache in looking back over 55 years of my career in physiotherapy practice. In the early days, while I was engaged in developing the best methods by which to treat my patients, triggered by my chance discovery with patient Mr Smith, I had no idea that the consequences of my work would be so profound. I recorded my observations over a 30-year period in practice and accumulated an enormous record of success using the diagnostic and treatment method described here. The notion of patient education and self-treatment grew naturally out of the therapy process.

The causes of common back problems had eluded medical experts for the past century and during the 1960s the term "non-specific back pain" became a catch-all diagnosis and a wide range of different treatments often conflicting became the standard offering by clinicians. My work initially offered me new options and with the significant successes achieved with my patients I wished more and more to share the methods that produced vastly better outcomes. My attempts to spread the word largely "fell on deaf eyes" so to speak; for 30 years there was simply enormous reluctance in the professions involved to recognize a simple, effective and inexpensive treatment.

"Centralizing pain" is now accepted worldwide as a probable indicator of disc pathology and is, to date, the most reliable predictor of a good outcome in treatment. There are now over 35 scientific papers on centralization and its reliability, and many more have examined centralization as a principle of diagnosis or treatment.

My books have supported my teaching and have spread knowledge of my treatment method even further. *Treat Your Own Back* has to date sold five million copies and is now available in 17 languages. It has become New Zealand's third-highest-selling book. The book was always meant to be an adjunct to the clinical treatment provided to patients. However, a study by Brian Undermann and colleagues published in 2004 showed that the book alone was effective in helping most with recurring and chronic back pain to decrease their own pain, reduce the frequency of, or eliminate entirely, their recurrent episodes of pain.

My professional life has been colourful and ultimately immensely rewarding, with the wide acceptance today of my work, the dimming in my memory of my setbacks and humiliations and, most importantly, the knowledge that all over the world people suffering with common physical low back pain are often now quickly and inexpensively treated, helped to understand the cause and shown how to treat themselves and respect their vital spines.

It has been very satisfying to receive enthusiastic accounts from clinicians throughout the world who are using my methods. I receive a continuous stream of correspondence from clinicians, stating how amazed they are with the simplicity of the concepts and their efficacy. Many report that they were very discouraged with the treatments that they previously had to offer their patients suffering back pain. When they learned of Mechanical Diagnosis and Therapy, their interest in treating spine patients was rejuvenated and saved them from abandoning their profession. It has been humbling to be a part of this revitalization.

Many of those who doubted, challenged and even set about discrediting or humiliating me have changed their minds about MDT or at least recognize it has a place in the options for treatment available. It has become irrefutably clear that the methods of diagnosis I had developed were valid, repeatable by others and effective in the hands of anyone taught by the Institute. What has remained equally true, however, is that while the method has been repeatedly verified in demonstration and practice, to date there is little formal recognition of the method in the international medical guidelines for the treatment of mechanical disorders of the spine. One can only wonder how many conclusive studies it takes to obtain such recognition. Am I disappointed? Yes I am, a little! But I have become used to that over time. I look forward to the day, and I am certain it will come, that such formal recognition is achieved. Lack of acknowledgement of the validity of MDT in the scientific literature on back pain is an indictment on those responsible for guiding spinal care. To the captains in the ivory towers I quote Oliver Cromwell addressing the "rump" Parliament in 1653: "You have been sat here too long for any good you have been doing. Depart I say, and let us have done with you. In the name of God, go!"

A few years ago, some 20 years after the Chicago Orthopaedic Association meeting in which John McCulloch brutally reduced me to pulp, I met him at a Spine Society meeting in Adelaide, where he walked up to me with outstretched hand and said, "Robin McKenzie, I owe you a great apology. You were right and I was wrong. I behaved very badly that day." Those were extraordinarily sweet words to hear.

It is, however, those who in so many various ways and over so many years have listened to me, come to believe in me, worked alongside me and supported me professionally who stand out in my mind and whose contributions and commitment and loyalty are as dear to me today as always. I hope I have named them all in the story I have told here – they have my deep gratitude always.

My family has been the truly strong spine in my life, supporting me in every possible way, living with my disappointments and tolerating my very frequent and lengthy absences overseas. Joy has always been a strong guide in so many ways. She never hesitates to tell me I am wrong and is more often than not correct when she does. She has infinite wisdom, is always considerate and caring of others, can see potential trouble long before it arrives and her judgement of character is impeccable. I would be lost without her.

Jan managed Spinal Publications for 25 years and oversaw the editing of several editions of my books. She has single-handedly reared and nurtured Simon, who is now studying for his Master's Degree in Forensic Science at Otago University. She is a member of the Board of Trustees of the McKenzie Institute International. For the past five years Jan has been assisting her partner Trevor Lawrence as his business manager. They plan to marry in early 2010.

David, who has been a sheep and cattle farmer for most of his life, is settling on a small holding near Waikanae with his partner Sharon. He was immediately at home as a young lad on *Sundance* and later became a passionate sailor on his own racing yacht *Reckless*. He has crewed in many races across the South Pacific Ocean, the Atlantic and the Mediterranean. They still sail his yacht *Reckless* when time allows.

Alistair also loved the boating adventures of his childhood and, after gaining experience in Southampton, England, became a builder and restorer of classical timber vessels and then later a marine surveyor. Alistair has raised his son Cahn, and daughter Tamar, who are both doing well in their final years at secondary school. They also go boating with their father whenever they get the chance.

Andrew is married to Diana and they have three children, Melanie, Jessica and Stuart, all still at school. After selling his farm in southern Hawkes Bay, he purchased a ten-acre lot near End Farm and over the past eight years has continued to plant trees and develop the property so that it now resembles a small park, that includes a lake and aviaries for doves and pigeons.

To my family, to Mr Smith and the patients who taught me all I know, and to Vert Mooney I give my most grateful thanks. To faculty and members of the McKenzie Institute branches worldwide I entrust you with task of developing the methods of MDT to their full potential. I know you will and I can now retire and leave it in your care. My thanks to you all.